MIDLIFE MYTHS, MENOPAUSE & BEYOND

HOW THE HEALTH CHOICES YOU MAKE TODAY, WILL DEFINE THE QUALITY OF THE REST OF YOUR LIFE

KAREN SPENCE

First published by Ultimate World Publishing 2025
Copyright © 2025 Karen Spence

ISBN

Paperback: 978-1-923425-71-2
Ebook: 978-1-923425-72-9

Cover design: Ultimate World Publishing
Layout and typesetting: Ultimate World Publishing
Editor: James Salmon
Cover Image Copyrights: Artush-Shutterstock.com

Ultimate World Publishing
Diamond Creek,
Victoria Australia 3089
www.writeabook.com.au

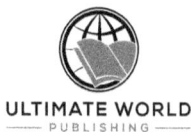

DEDICATION

To my mum, my sisters and brothers.

My family is everything to me.

To my husband Ivan and our daughter Rebecca.

There are no words I could write that would accurately describe my love for you.

Thank you both for making me a better person.

DISCLAIMER

The content of this book is drawn from many sources. They include years of research and women's health-related study. During my years as a health, weight-loss and fitness coach I have specifically focussed on the requirements of women over the age of 40.

Through personal interactions with middle-aged, peri-post menopausal women, I was able to unravel many of the tribulations of reaching middle age, whilst simultaneously going through the menopausal phases myself.

The information contained in this book is not intended to replace any advice or recommendations given to you by a medical professional regarding any specific ailments or conditions you may have.

CONTENTS

INTRODUCTION

I felt compelled to write this book to reach women who may feel like I once did. Like most other people, I endured a number of challenges in my life. The message I want to share with you is that you can overcome these challenges, no matter how hard they seem or to what depth they push you down.

Although the phases of menopause are featured throughout the book, this book is as much about everyday life as a middle-aged woman, and the ups-and-downs we have lived through to shape us into who we are today.

You can make peace with the past and with people who may have hurt you, and not let unwanted memories continue to cloud or influence your life, now or in your future. You can change your narrative and adopt a more positive and purposeful outlook.

Of course, the challenges, difficulties and successes you have encountered throughout your life have played a massive part in shaping who you are - your attitude, your opinion, your choices and of course life has its curveballs. But most of what you encounter is yours to change, if it is no longer serving who you are now or who you feel you need to be. You can't change past experiences; they are what they are. However, you can decide how you continue to deal with them in your mind, what lessons you will learn from them and how you let them influence your thoughts, decisions and actions.

Each phase of my life has, without doubt, been an iterative process. I didn't know that's what was happening at the time, but looking back I can see how the person I am now, evolved from those periods of repeated uncertainty, difficulty, success and then growth. There have been many versions of me.

You are not defined by a past or a bad experience, a toxic relationship or perceived failures. And you are certainly not defined by other people's opinions of you either then or now.

In writing this book I would like every woman who reads it to look at her life, assess her state of contentment and review her aspirations. I sincerely hope that you are happy and you wouldn't change a thing. If you're not, only you have the power to make the changes to create opportunities. Only you can overhaul the areas of your life you are not fully satisfied with - including your health and your relationships - and anything that stands in the way of your self-preservation and your pursuit of happiness.

You have the right to have a fulfilling and healthful life, for all your life. Don't let anyone tell you otherwise or tell you it's not what you deserve. You do. Preserve the essence of who you are but do what's right for you. Compromise but don't give in. You have the right to live your life on your own terms. It's not going to please everyone in your life. But it's not about them - it's about you.

I say in the book that you don't have to step on or over people to achieve what you want for yourself, and you don't. However, you may need to ask them to step aside or just walk around them if they stand in your way. You need to continue your life's journey uninhibited.

Take from the book what resonates with you. Make changes in your life if you need to, and let people go if you feel it's a necessary step for you to keep moving forward.

Middle age is still only half-way through your life. Take control of the second half. Live it on your terms.

CHAPTER 1

WELL HELLO MIDDLE AGE - HOW THE HELL DID YOU GET HERE?

"Ageing is not 'lost youth' but a new
stage of opportunity and strength."
Betty Friedan, Activist

BORN A WOMAN

Right now, millions of women around the world are treading the same path as generations of women before them. Regardless of country, colour, beliefs, social background or financial status, women become biologically equal when they reach middle age and menopause. The effects of changing hormones on a woman's physical, emotional and mental wellbeing, and the symptoms experienced, are all part of the natural ageing process and do not discriminate.

On the approach to middle age, many women can feel lost in the changes occurring, not least because the symptoms of middle age and the phases of menopause are not always visible. Your body is going through a major biological transformation. Those around you don't understand, or they don't try to understand, choosing to believe, 'if it can't be seen it isn't happening', as a reason for not acknowledging or playing down your discomfort.

An effect of this lack of understanding and acknowledgement is that women can feel isolated and misunderstood. These factors have contributed to middle-aged women becoming the fastest growing group in depression and anxiety statistics.

You might be just turning 40 and realising - to your horror - that society now deems you to be middle-aged. You may be struggling with the idea yourself, whilst battling the discomforting traits of perimenopause - wondering when the hell it's going to stop and you will start to feel better.

If you are into your 50s or early 60s you will have already gone through menopause, and having ticked that box you may be wondering what happens next. What is your purpose in life, now that so many changes have occurred to bring you to exactly where you are at this juncture.

A bit of an eye-opener for me was the realisation that middle-aged women are seemingly invisible in society. Many examples led me to this conclusion, but the most overt one was when a few years ago I was viewing an age-health chart. This chart highlighted issues and conditions commonly experienced by women and had them listed under two headings - 'Adult - 25-45' and 'Elderly - 65+'. I remember thinking, "Hang on a minute! What about us, the in-betweenies, those who are 46–64-year-olds? Where do we fit in?"

It's like, we are not young so we can't be counted there, we're not yet old, so we're not counted there - we're just hanging around in a virtual waiting room - waiting until we have accumulated enough years to be called forward to be placed conveniently into the 'old-people' box, because apparently, society will then know how to deal with us. Once we get a new title of ill or infirm, alone and lonely, dependent on others, we can then be referred to specific service providers to look after us.

For the record, middle age is considered to be between 40 – 60 or 45 – 65 depending on the source. Regardless, the actual numbers are not important because your body is doing the counting all on its own. During this time much happens to a woman, physically, mentally and emotionally. It can simultaneously have both wonderfully positive and crushingly negative effects, across all aspects of her life.

How you deal with this phase of your life is entirely up to you. By that I mean you have a choice. You may consider that where you are today was pre-determined by your upbringing, your relationships, your job or your partner. You may be really happy with how your life evolved and be totally satisfied. Alternatively, you may be in the group of women who are not entirely happy with their life and believe there was nothing that could have been done that would have made any difference. Conversely, you may be aware that you could have done things differently and created a different outcome - but you didn't.

None of that matters now. Your life is not in your past. It is right here, right now, and this is where your focus needs to be. Prepare and plan for what comes next, and into the future. No one can do this for you. If you want to change aspects of your life, you are the one who needs to make the effort to make it happen.

It might be difficult and uncomfortable at times, but believe in yourself.

'Believe you can, and you're halfway there.'
Theodore Roosevelt

PERPLEXING PUBERTY

Let's go back in time and recall the dim and distant memory of puberty and 'becoming a woman', with all the sweet naivety of being a young teenager, believing that you are now 'grown-up'. From the elation of 'oh yay I have boobs!' to the misery of 'oh no, I have a period!' I remember both vividly.

It is said that people always remember their 'first' of everything. Do you recall when you got your first bra? I do. I was always a skinny kid, and I was so excited at the first fledgling buds that were sprouting on my otherwise completely flat body. I asked my mum if I could have a bra. She laughed and asked me what I was going to put in it. She humoured me though and bought me my first bra. It was a size 30AA, the smallest size available. She sewed the cups smaller so it fitted me. I was really pleased that now when I got changed for school PT sessions, I no longer had to suffer the embarrassment of being the only girl in class still wearing a vest. Although if I'm honest, I was still made fun of. I didn't mind though - I had a bra!

My first period was not such a proud moment. In fact, it was mortifying. My parents were separated by this time. Mum had moved out temporarily leaving us at home with Dad. He was an alcoholic, in poor health and unable to look after himself, never mind four kids under 12.

I got my first period during this time, and I didn't know what to do. I was too embarrassed to tell my dad… I mean, he was a man… and my dad! I just cried a lot. My two elder sisters were both married and had left home, and we didn't have a phone, so I couldn't contact them.

My 16-year-old brother was still at home, but there was not a chance in hell I was going to tell him. Dad saw my distress, and he sat me down. Although I was too embarrassed to tell him, he eventually figured it out. He gave me some money and told me to go to the chemist, tell the woman in the shop what had happened, and she would give me what I needed. My dad was unable to cope with many things in his too-short life, but he handled this situation admirably. He was so out of his comfort zone, poor sod.

For most women, the raging hormones of puberty is followed in later years by the raging hormones of pregnancy and childbirth, multiple times for some. The years pass, and just when we think we are starting to regain control of our life and body, we are suddenly 30-something, and the whole fluctuating hormone thing starts happening all over again.

Now our hormones are not the bad guys we sometimes make them out to be. They are a vital component of all aspects of our health and wellbeing. Certain hormones influence the essential workings of your body, as well as your behaviour and your mood. When your hormones are balanced, so are you. If your hormones are not balanced, neither are you.

After the age of 35, your ovaries start to produce less oestrogen, the hormone responsible for preparing your body for conception and birth. This is the signal that you are approaching middle age and the chance of a healthy pregnancy is significantly reduced. Your body responds by making it more difficult for you to conceive.

Everyone is different, but around this time, women enter the perimenopausal phase that many consider to be puberty in reverse, same mood swings, irritability and heightened emotions. As the years go on there is the added discourtesy of sleepless nights, hot flushes, and needing to pee more often!

ECHOES OF YESTERYEAR

Let's go back even further. Back to when you were a child. If you were a child in the 50s your mum was likely a housewife or worked in a female-specific role. She would have been the primary caregiver to the children in your household and responsible for shopping, cooking and cleaning and other areas of day-to-day domesticity.

Dads generally were not overly involved in domestic activities at that time. They were considered the main financial provider given that men were the higher income earners or just paid more than women, even for doing the same job. At this time, women were still considered unreliable employees as it was deemed inevitable that they would leave a job to get married and have children.

That said, changes had begun years before when during WWII, women stepped-up to fill the gaps in the workforce and perform the roles of men who had gone off to war. This brought about a huge social shift and a rise in the diversity of roles for women, who were now being employed in what had previously been considered men's jobs.

Many men didn't return from the war; of those who did, a large number were injured or disabled. This prolonged the significant labour force shortages that women continued to fill through the 50s. As economic stability returned, this became an issue. Women didn't want to relinquish their employment, but men were returning to the workforce, and young men were entering the employment market for the first time. Women were reluctant to revert to their former 'stay-at-home' role and were often accused of 'stealing men's jobs', but it was a massive turning point for women's independence.

However, even greater change was on the horizon. The swinging 60s came around bringing the Beatles, Woodstock, flower power, free love and of course, burning your bra. Women growing up in the 60s were, unbeknown to them, living through the beginning of massive societal change.

From the 60s era of sex, drugs and rock and roll to disco-dancing through the 70s in a blur of bell-bottoms, hot pants and glam rock and then into the 80s with big hair, ripped jeans and punk. Through it all came a change in women's attitude to themselves and their role in society.

Women more tenaciously stood up for equal rights and equal opportunities, striving to be liberated from male dependency and end male domination in certain roles, whilst increasing their influence on social and political platforms.

So many gains were made over those years, which makes it all the more astonishing that today, women are still fighting for fairness and inclusivity in many areas of society.

When you were growing up through those years, in your teens and twenties - did you have ideas about what kind of life you would have, where you would go and who you would become, when you were older? And in those youthful years, what age did you consider to be middle-aged and old? Now you've reached the crossroads, is it what you expected? Has your life turned out as you planned, hoped or thought it would?

The funny thing is, girls born in the mid-80s, who no doubt once looked upon women aged in their 40s as old, are now in their mid-40s themselves - and no doubt they don't feel old at all. Nonetheless, today's young teens and 20-somethings will consider them to be old. The point is, perceptions of what it is to look, feel and be middle-aged is different for everyone, depending on which rung of life's ladder you currently sit.

It's cathartic when those of us who are middle-aged and older look at younger people just starting out in the independent world. We know just what it feels like. For us it seems like yesterday. Memories come flooding back. Many of us will recall all the plans we had ourselves at their age.

I was told a story of a preschooler who, when asked what she thought she would be like when she was 40, she said "I probably won't be able to walk properly, and I'll be nearly dead". I hope for her sake that when she is 40, she will chuckle if reminded she once said that.

Do you ever wonder, if you had done things differently or made different choices, just how differently your life may have turned out? There are those who say that your fate is pre-determined. I am not one of those people. Yes, some things happen, and you wonder how or why it did and if fate lent a hand. But I believe you set down your own pathway, you create your own luck, and you contrive your own opportunities. So, when that door of opportunity opens, you are ready to walk right through it, grasp what is being offered with both hands and make something of it.

I'm not suggesting even for one second that plenty of women are not totally happy and content with the life they have created, whether it is as a high-level executive or as a stay-at-home mum. If a woman is at one with the choices she has made, regardless of what those choices are, that is exactly what striving for and achieving happiness is. High level ambition is not something everyone needs to have, but everyone does need a sense of purpose.

On the other side of the coin, I know from the many women I have spoken to, that some look back on their life and have regrets that they didn't do the things they planned or achieve more than they have. Some feel resentful because life got in the way or took an unexpected turn and prevented them from fulfilling a dream or reaching a goal. Maybe you lacked the courage to go after something you wanted, or the circumstances weren't right; it wasn't the right time, there was not enough money, you had dependents, young or old. There are those who will believe that it's now too late.

If this is you, I'm here to tell you that it isn't too late. And the reason it's not too late, is because it's never too late - to follow a dream or achieve a goal. We're not talking about climbing Everest or skydiving (unless you want to), but everyday goals that contribute to feelings of satisfaction and accomplishment. You can continue to seek out new adventures or learn something new that will contribute to your sense of purpose and achievement. Nothing is stopping you - other than yourself.

You will have learned throughout your life that the reasons that influence whether we do something or not, come up time and time again. Much of the time they are just excuses for not doing things we are too scared to do for fear of rejection or failure; we make ourselves believe they are justifiable. When an opportunity presents itself, take it. Just say yes - and then work the rest out. If you truly want it, you'll find a way to achieve it. Be accountable to yourself and not beholden to others.

When the actress Helen Mirren was asked what she didn't do when she was younger that she wished she had done, she said she wished she had "told more people to fuck off", demonstrating that you can keep it simple and achievable with little room for misunderstanding! When I think back on the people I allowed to influence my life through the years, that I really shouldn't have, I imagine it would have been very satisfying to say that to them.

Don't hold yourself back and don't let anyone else hold you back. Do what you need to do, invoke your freedom of choice and forge your way ahead.

Our life choices and our experiences up to middle age, both good and bad, have shaped us into the people we are today. My aim in this book is to encourage and guide you to embrace middle age in the same enthusiastic way you embraced being in your teens, twenties and thirties.

You can still stamp your mark on society, despite the notion that continues to define middle-aged women as having served their purpose, faded into the background and dropped down to a rung of insignificance on society's ladder of relevance.

Reaching middle age is a celebration of new possibilities, a time for reflection and reassessment of your purpose, and for continuing growth.

BECOMING WHO YOU ARE

We all have a different story of how we came to be where we are today, and much of that story was moulded in the era we were born, the society we were raised in, and the kind of home life we grew up in.

I was born in the 50s, the middle child of seven children, with an alcoholic father who couldn't hold down a job and a mum who did the very best she could to hold us all together. I didn't understand or appreciate until many years later how difficult her life had been, and that much of the time she was barely keeping herself together.

My mum once told me that she could have achieved much more in her life, but given her circumstances, her options had been limited.

In 1949, Mum became pregnant to an American GI stationed near where she lived in the UK. He had wanted her to go back to the States with him, but she didn't want to leave her family. She gave birth to my eldest sister, and although the father was told of the birth of his daughter, he never contacted my mum, and they had no further communication.

When my mum and dad met, my sister was 9 months old. They married after a relatively short courtship. Although not uncommon during and after the war, an illegitimate child was still scandalous and gossip-worthy. In the early years of their marriage, Mum had described Dad as a gentleman – he always treated her well and respectfully. What became apparent as the years ticked by - and the number of children grew - was that Dad became increasingly unable to cope, and was spending more and more time and what little money we had at the pub.

None of the family can recall first-hand the dynamics of their relationship that led to the eventual breakdown of the marriage, but I know Mum was unhappy for most of it. There was never any money and Mum struggled to feed and clothe us all. We all wore 'hand-me-downs'. I remember her saying, "When poverty comes in through the window, love flies out of the door". Mum had a difficult and unfulfilled adult life that started with misguided, but understandable decisions made in her early twenties, a 20-year marriage, the majority of the latter years unhappily, whilst working and raising seven children.

Mum had already met someone else when she and my dad separated. I didn't know this at the time, or in fact until he moved into our house. She thought she had found love, but he was no more husband or father material than my dad had been. He was also a drinker, and although Dad had volatile outbursts, he was passive most of the time, whereas this one was a violent drunk and I despised him. Had he been a decent man and made Mum happy, and had he been a good stepfather to the four of us still at home, I would have been happy for her. But he was none of those things, and I hate that she was as disillusioned as ever and never truly found happiness.

We were fortunate that all seven siblings looked out for each other, especially the ones younger than ourselves. I believe our upbringing had a profound effect on each of us in different ways. We grew up to be very close. We supported each other through some tough times, and we are testament to what strength and pride the love of a family can bring. We're a little bruised and scarred - but we were never broken.

Sometimes you have to dig deep to find the reasons your life turned out the way it did. What influences, hardships or experiences shaped your thinking. It might have been one decision you made or an accumulation of circumstances that steered your path.

Many women no doubt had a definitive plan, some would have drifted into a certain lifestyle whilst others ran headlong into it with a 'whatever will be, will be' attitude. Some are dealt a cruel hand that may have dictated their life-path - sometimes events along the way can take away your capacity to choose freely.

There have likely been times of great happiness and achievement in your life, and undoubtedly, moments of intense sadness and disappointment. You might believe that some of these events continue to shape your life, and it's likely that they do.

Nonetheless, and all raw emotion aside, they are events in moments in time. It is how you dealt with those moments, good or bad, that would have had the biggest impact on your future endeavours. It is what you allowed those events to teach you that counts. Whether you walked away from them feeling empowered or bitter, defeated or determined, broken or regenerated, it's the emotions you experienced that will have influenced you and played a part in crafting your outlook and pathway in life.

If you're struggling with negativities from your past, it's time to lay them to rest. If past disappointments or mistakes are stopping you from living the life you want to live now, it's time to wipe the slate clean and choose the direction of your future.

You may think it's not possible to change some things in your life now, but how do you know unless you try? Sometimes you decide things can't be changed because you lack the courage to change it, or to walk away and let go of things in your life that are no longer serving your best interests.

We are going to explore all these things throughout this book. I will challenge you to analyse your thought processes, question the validity of your decisions and consider alternative points of view. This can guide you towards the answers you seek and provide clarity on your journey through middle age and beyond.

CHAPTER 2

CARE, CONFORM, COMPROMISE, CONTROL

BORN TO CARE

As women we are deemed to be naturally caring and nurturing souls, given that we are the bearer of children and regarded as the gentler sex. I'm not going to cast aspersions about the validity of the 'naturally nurturing' label because there is evidence to prove that we are biologically predisposed to this.

However, there are some schools of thought that suggest that the continuing idea of 'woman, the natural caregiver' is used more as a social construct to support the gender-biased ideal of the role of a woman, in what is still a male-dominated society. The traditional perception and expectations are that women care more; therefore, they must be better at looking after children and the elderly and be more domestically inclined.

Over the last 50 years it cannot be denied that the gender divide has narrowed. Although women are still viewed as the primary caregivers and generally tend to the domestic affairs in a household, modern men appear more comfortable with domesticity in a way that would make their grandfathers and for some, their fathers, shake their head in disbelief.

There is evidence abound that women are just as capable as men in most things, and that men are just a capable as women. Whether it's raising a child or working in a mine. It doesn't matter who's bigger, stronger or smarter, both sexes have the capacity and capability to learn a job or a skill and do it as well as each other.

CARING FOR YOURSELF

Whilst caring for others may come naturally to most women, caring for themselves does not; women will put the needs of those they love before their own needs.

Several studies show that, although women may neither ask nor expect anything in return, it's important for them to know that the people they care for - especially their significant other, parents, children, friends and close work colleagues - also care for and appreciate them.

Many women feel underappreciated and indeed they are. You may be able to relate to this and have felt this way at some point in your adult life.

Women can also get overly concerned about making decisions they perceive others will judge them for. They may wish to pursue an interest, change their job or leave an unhappy or unhealthy relationship. They hesitate to decide because they fear the reaction of others and need external affirmation that it's okay.

This kind of insecurity in their own power to make the right decision for themselves could be residual of years spent undervalued or overlooked in the workplace, or from being underappreciated and taken for granted at home.

It's not wrong or unhealthy to care what others think about you or the decisions you make for yourself - unless you care obsessively. If you do, this suggests deeper issues of insecurity and low self-worth. If you allow this to impact your ability to think and decide independently, over time you will find yourself seeking validation for even the smallest of decisions, which could lead to a significant impact on your mental health.

There's nothing wrong in asking those you trust for an opinion. Sometimes though, others have their own agenda and can influence you in a way that brings you to a decision that isn't the best one for you.

I was talking recently with one of my clients about her early life. She got married and had two daughters whilst she was still in her mid-teens. When the marriage ended, she chose to focus on her children and never entered into another meaningful relationship.

The children grew-up, left home, married and had children of their own. She started to work part-time and looked after her grandchildren a few days a week, and for some evenings and weekends, whilst their parents worked and socialised.

Now approaching 50, her life and her needs have started to change. She's planning to return to full-time employment; she has met a new partner and is enjoying being in a relationship again. She feels she is emotionally and socially ready to start living her own life. She spent her teens and adult life being Mum and then Grandma, both roles she loves dearly. However, she now feels she is in the right place at the right time to create a life for herself - for the first time in her life.

She is so happy. Her children are not. They had a long list of arguments. Who would look after their kids while they work and socialise? Who would take their kids for the weekend when they wanted to get away for a break? What was the point in her going to back to work full-time when another grandbaby is due soon, and she would need to look after them too? And wait for it... why was she even bothering to make changes to her life at her age?

She cares very much what they think and was feeling terrible - worrying if this made her an awful mother and grandmother. She doesn't want it to harm her relationship with her daughters and grandchildren. They are heaping on the guilt and it's working, but she's also very upset that her children can't be happy for her, and she feels torn.

She acknowledges that she allowed the situation to unfold over the years. She had felt it was her purpose to guide and help her children in a way that no one had done for her. But she also believes she has fulfilled that purpose. I was pleased when she told me she had let them know to work out alternative arrangements for when she had her own plans, and that there should be no expectation that she would be available on demand.

She is ready to take back her own life and has decided not to let anyone else's expectations of her take priority over the ones she now has for herself.

You can't live your life serving other people's expectations of you. The only expectations you should be striving to live up to are your own, and ultimately, the final decision is yours to make, in your own best interest. Your mental health is as important as your physical and emotional health. Keep the balance.

You can't be everything to everyone - so just be yourself. If people don't like it or criticise you for it, you need to question the depth of your relationship with them, and if and why their opinion matters.

Every woman will grow at her own pace, and when the time is right, she will be drawn to a new purpose. It may happen only once, or it may happen many times over her lifetime. And that's okay, it's allowed! You have every right to change aspects of your life if you want to, without fear and without guilt.

Sadly, guilt is a very powerful tool that is wielded through manipulation, even by those we love and who love us. We concede because we care about not hurting other people's feelings, and don't want others to think badly of us - especially not our family. Women find it hard to say no. We tend to drift along with situations we don't really want to be part of, out of obligation and because it's expected.

Many of us were raised this way. But it doesn't mean it has to stay that way, or that you can't start making changes now.

When someone tells me they are being taken for granted, I ask them why they are allowing it to happen. Push back. They are only doing it because you accept the way they behave towards you. Don't let them.

> *"No-one can make you feel inferior*
> *without your consent."*
> *Eleanor Roosevelt*

Being there for someone because they need emotional support is done naturally and unhesitatingly for those you care about. It is a way to show your love and support. If you are a naturally giving person, never change who you are, but also don't let that spill over to allow your good intentions and kind heart to be taken for granted.

TAUGHT TO CONFORM

Women who are now in their middle years were taught at home and at school what would be expected of them in later life. We dutifully conformed to the way of the world at that time. Men too. I don't know about you, but at school I learned typing, sewing and domestic science (cooking), and the boys got to do the good stuff, like woodwork and metalwork. I wanted to do that, but I wasn't allowed to because I was a girl. Apparently, I wouldn't be needing those skills.

My daughter laughed when I told her this story and recalled the occasion she came home to find her dad and I talking at the front of the property. Dad was going out to buy some new cotton spools for the sewing machine and Velcro to finish a sewing job he was doing, and I was saying goodbye to him with my chainsaw still slung across my shoulder from taking down some trees in the yard.

However, back in the day I conformed as required and left school at 16 to go to secretarial college to learn shorthand and clerical work. I knew I wanted more than that - to see more and do more. So, I did what any small, skinny, naïve, unworldly 17-year-old girl would do. I joined the military. Well you do, don't you? My mum said she would give me three months before I gave it up and came home. Sorry Mum, but it was the best decision I could have made. I served for 15 years and I loved that life.

That said, when I joined the British Army in 1975, all females were enlisted into the Women's Royal Army Corp (WRAC). Despite being 'in the Army', the only careers offered were support and domestic roles; cook, communications, clerical, driving, stewardess.

I left the Army in July 1990. By April 1992, the WRAC had been disbanded, and women's roles were integrated into the once male-only Corps and Regiments. Previously unavailable employment roles were opened up to women for the first time, and it was widely believed that the integration would equalise opportunities.

Despite that, by 1997 still only 47% of the roles in the Army were available to women. Incredibly, it wasn't until 2018 that all roles in the British Army were finally opened for women to apply for. It wasn't that women didn't want to do these roles, or weren't qualified or capable of doing them, they just weren't allowed. (All statistics and dates courtesy of the British Legion.)

External perceptions still dictate what women are, or are not, capable of doing - particularly as they get older. On a positive note, fewer middle-aged women are inclined to put up with other people's shit anymore and be dictated to. The 'shut up and put up' days are diminishing rapidly, and women of all ages believe in their right to pursue any career or interests they choose. There is no time or age limit on this - if there is a job you want and you know you can do it, no matter your age, go get it.

You can make decisions that can literally change your life. How often do you say to yourself, "I wish I'd done that or gone there"? What's stopping you doing it now? There may well be physical or financial limitations to some of the things you want to do, but don't use that as an excuse to do nothing.

The odds on you winning the lottery are not good, so don't be waiting for that to happen before you realise a dream. In any case, not everything worth doing needs lots of money or youthful fitness levels, or even skill. If necessary, set new, smaller and achievable goals, and see how good it feels to once again start ticking off the boxes on your 'things I'd like to do' list.

Positive Compromise

Compromising is not conforming. Compromise is about mutual concessions, give and take, agreed outcomes by each giving ground to the other person to reach a fair and equally favourable conclusion. If one person ends up conceding more than they are comfortable with, they may become hostile, resentful and bitter.

This is true for everyone, in every type of relationship. Sometimes you might decide to give a bit more to help somebody and if you are comfortable with that, it's okay. It's not unreasonable to ask others to do the same for you, to accommodate your growth, your change in circumstances or simply your choices.

When you decide to make changes to your life, the considerate thing to do would be to assess what impact the changes you make may have on those around you. You would expect the same courtesy. That said, you can't let other people's agenda influence your decisions if they are only self-serving. If someone is concerned that the personal decisions and life changes you make will negatively impact on them, it might just be because they consider their needs to be greater than yours. Don't buy into it. Talk it through, compromise where necessary, but pursue what's right for you. Your life. Your decision.

Your destiny is yours to shape, your choices are yours to make in line with what you believe, what you value, and what you want for yourself. Once you have figured out the direction you want to take, start moving towards it.

You don't have to step on or over anyone to achieve it - but you may have to ask them to step aside or go around them to bring about the outcome that you want for yourself.

Being kind is different again. That's your heart talking. Don't let people take your kindness for granted. Kindness is an underused commodity in the modern, fast-paced, high-tech shambles that is humanity. So be the kindness in what can sometimes be a shitty, violent, unpredictable and uncaring world.

Kindness is yours to give, give it freely, receive it humbly and spread it everywhere. And sure, your kind and positive attitude is bound to piss off some miserable sod - but do it anyway!

COMFORTABLY IN CONTROL

We talk about taking control of our life and I'm totally on board with that. I do, however, wonder what 'control' looks like to different people. Sometimes I think the term 'control' sounds too rigid, too unbending.

Doing things on your own terms is healthy and admirable. Needing to have absolute control over everything in your life could steer you towards being uncompromising and inflexible, bitter and disappointed - and not much fun to live, work or socialise with. Some things will never be yours to control, no matter how much you'd like to. Life just isn't like that.

To quote an old adage, 'Change what you can, accept what you can't'. It is up to you to exercise your own power to accept that you can't control everything and come to terms with that before you let your emotions dictate your actions and drive your decision-making. This is not a failing; this is self-awareness.

Pushing yourself to your limits to achieve your goals can be extremely satisfying. But knowing your limitations is a strength that will be your buffer between becoming frustrated and disillusioned with your efforts. Being self-aware can help you to un-litter your brain and direct your energy towards the things you can do, the things you can change and highlight what you need to let go of. This will allow you to focus and pursue a healthier, more productive life-path.

CHAPTER 3

STOP EATING THE HYPE - STOP BELIEVING THE LIES

IN THE OLD DAYS...

Historically, and I mean way back, women lived in a much more unequal society than we do now. Throughout history women have asserted their power and influence by using their looks and body as a way of surviving in a world, socially and financially, traditionally or culturally, controlled by men.

Women behaved and dressed in the manner of how a woman should look, that befitted the expectations of the day. In the Victorian era, women went to extreme measures of discomfort to enhance their womanly features. From corsets that squished the waistline until boobs were pushed out and lungs were so restricted that she fainted, to bustles fitted under the dress at the back to make their behind look bigger, as well as overly painted faces and outrageous wigs.

Although the sit down, don't speak and look pretty days may be (almost) gone, the practice of women using the means available to them to enhance and accentuate their body and face is alive and kicking - and still to extremes. Except now, instead of just using clothing and make-up to enhance the body and face, it is Botox, boob jobs and butt-lifts.

Why is it I wonder, that so many women go to excessive and sometimes drastic measures, to get a certain look. It's as though women of all ages are still conforming to those same societal expectations of what is considered attractive and feel duty bound to comply.

I can't help but wonder why young women especially, choose to look so fake, over-pouted and over-painted, going to great lengths it seems, to look like everyone else in their peer group. It looks like every young woman is an expert make-up artist and they are always 'camera ready', looking completely flawless at any time of day or night. It must be exhausting!

I have also wondered why middle-aged women opt for excessive face altering procedures, seemingly to make themselves look younger. Interestingly, the reasons women give are based more on their wish to improve their emotional and psychological wellness rather than physical enhancement - in other words, feel better about themselves. They are keen to slow down the ageing process not necessarily regarding how they look, but to recover the 'feelings' of their younger self.

The issue middle-aged women often ponder, is that they don't feel any different in their 40s, 50s and 60s than they did in their 20s and 30s. However, the face they see in the mirror, does not reflect the person they feel they still are in their heart and mind.

I believe that it is this disconnect that causes older women to attempt to balance how they feel and how they look. It pushes them to take advantage of the cosmetic and surgical measures readily available, to enable them to do that. But how far do you go? What is enough and what is too much?

INJECTION OF DELUSION

I find myself at odds around the subject of cosmetic and surgical enhancements. I feel conflicted when I see a woman who has quite obviously undergone excessive procedures. Botox treatments for example. Botox is a muscle paralysis toxin that, when injected into the muscles in your face, causes them to relax and smooth out and reduce wrinkles. The common side effects, the ones considered less serious, like double vision, difficulty swallowing, breathing or speaking, and muscle weakness, is likely considered acceptable to the women who have it, to achieve the desired effect.

The problem is, to keep the look, you must keep having top-ups. According to the Mayo Clinic, 'the long-lasting cosmetic use of botulinum toxin (Botox) can trigger permanent changes in facial expression and an expressionless, mask-like face'. You have only to look at the film industry and other celebrity figures to see this is fact.

Injectables are big business. You can inject just about any body part. Dermal fillers to plump your cheeks and pout your lips. Injections for your butt cheeks to make your bum more shapely. If you were a man, you would have the option to have a penis enlargement using fat grafting. You wish I hadn't told you that don't you? Let's never speak of it again!

There are of course other reasons for this than wanting to recapture youthful times. Every woman is different, and her reasons for the choices she makes are hers alone.

Perhaps some women who have these treatments do it to boost their confidence, as a power play, or simply as a mask to hide insecurities. Or maybe it's none of those things?

Regardless, I find it difficult to fathom why someone would voluntarily allow toxic substances to be injected into them for non-medical reasons. For me it just begs the question "Why the fuck would you do that!" I've kicked the hornet's nest haven't I?

If reading this, you are someone who has opted for procedures, it isn't my intention to offend you. If you are happy and confident with the decisions you have made and how it makes you look and feel, my opinion and that of everyone else should not matter a fig to you. You no doubt have your reasons and… yeah, I still sound judgy don't I? Moving on.

It's no surprise that older women are tempted down this path though. Everywhere you look you are bombarded with how you can improve your looks - how to achieve a toned body at 50, the poutiest lips at 55, plumped-out cheeks at 60, the most fabulous eyelashes at 65 and wrinkle-free skin at 70. All these companies need to do is agitate your insecurities sufficiently and they have you primed, ready and willing to spend a shit-tonne of money.

Alternatively, you can do as they do in the ads to achieve that flawless photo - use one of the many filtering techniques to slim and smooth you to within an inch of your life. It's a good time to remind you that in real life, the women you see in the photo ads don't look at all in life as they do in the photos.

Age doesn't seem to be a factor in who is eating up the hype that is served up ad nauseum. Our lives are now so completely saturated with what we need to do before and after the age of 40, what we should no longer be doing, what to eat and what to wear, to look and feel 'young, slim and beautiful'. The underlying message is designed to lure you to tap into your vulnerabilities and have you comparing yourself with others.

MANIPULATIVE MARKETING

I saw an ad recently that wasn't even a subtle message, it was a straight-out order. "Women over 50! Stop doing (this) now!" I see an ad like this and I think, "Get stuffed!" I'm just so over this in-your-face claptrap.

You can't escape it though. It's everywhere: magazines, television, Instagram, Facebook, TikTok, text messages, emails. All are attempting to brainwash you into believing you need to meet the exacting standards of how it is perceived a woman should look and behave, to be noticed, considered attractive, the right shape, an acceptable weight, popular and relevant in today's society.

The list is endless. We're shown photos of women who look 25 but are supposedly 55 - and all because they have been using this new, age defying face-cream! Give us a break. It's photoshopped. We're middle-aged, not stupid!

We have all been influenced by intensive marketing at some time or another. You see something online, in a magazine or a store that you liked the look of - a face cream or make-up, a weight-loss product, an item of clothing. It looks and sounds really good, and the model looks great. But it's hard to know anymore what's real, what is fake or filtered, and what is just a downright money-generating scam.

Nevertheless, you read the write-up of the amazing benefits and what it could do for you. You read the amazing testimonials of 'satisfied clients' who have used it with 'life-changing' results.

You had never seen or heard of this product before, but you liked what you saw, were convinced it was just what you needed, and you bought it. That's the power of marketing. It's all around us every hour of every day. We all succumb to it. The beauty and weight loss industries have thrived on our gullibility.

I say all of that with a little exaggeration in my disdain. I buy moisturisers, hand creams etc that are marketed as appropriate for my age-group. Do they work any better than any of the others? I don't know. The marketing tells me the ingredients are perfect for my aging, wrinkly skin. I know I like some more than others, but I can honestly say that I am never expecting it to make me wrinkle free or look 10 years younger. Damn you marketing!

I saw a headline on a news page that read:

"5 Things you MUST do to keep people thinking you are younger than your age."

I am always intrigued when I see this sort of title, seemingly aimed at informing middle-aged women that it's not socially acceptable to look your actual age.

I started to read the new wonder methods for eternal youth. This is what it said:

'Tip number one - fill your mouth with coconut oil and pump your cheeks in and out." What the fuck! Seriously!

Just the thought of doing that triggered my gag reflexes. Am I so concerned with people thinking I look younger than my age that I'm going to risk choking on coconut oil?

And no, I can't share the other 4 tips because I skimmed over the detail. If the first one was an indication of the gruelling measures I would have to go to for smooth baby-arse skin at my age, I shall embrace my wrinkles with immense pride and considerable relief.

And then there's beef fat. Apparently, this is the key to 'glass skin', recommended to anyone with wrinkly skin. Testimonials read "Everyone says I look 10 years younger" and "Beef Fat changed my life!" So, there you have it. Your life is worthless and all you need to change it is gargle coconut oil and spread beef fat on your face. Somebody save us!

Do all women at the age of 40, on reaching the dreaded number that is considered middle age, suddenly feel the need to look like they did in their 20s? No of course not. However, most of us are likely to have been using at least the basic cosmetic products since our teens; make-up, make-up remover, cleanser and moisturiser, in some brand or other, because we cared how we looked and took pride in our appearance.

I remember when I bought my first products. I was 17, I'd just started earning a weekly wage, buying clothes and wearing make-up. In those early days I would remove my make-up, which consisted of eyeshadow, mascara and lipstick, with baby oil, clean my face with baby lotion and then wash my face with soap and water. That was until a skincare representative from a beauty company visited our Army camp to speak to us ladies about her company's products, that would save us from having prune faces before the age of 20.

And so it began. My first exposure to being influenced by beauty industry marketing! It was here I was introduced to purpose-made products and bought make-up remover, cleanser, toner and moisturiser. I'd never spent money on anything like that before and I felt proper grown up! I can tell you that I was most definitely not buying it to look younger. At 17 I barely looked 12 as it was!

However, being influenced to buy those items that day was the start of a life-long self-care habit (just what marketers love) of cleaning my face properly, every day. It's a basic routine that stayed with me since the days of not wanting pimply skin on my face. Has doing this made a difference to how my skin looks now? Maybe, we'll never know.

What then, is the difference between self-care, self-pride and self-obsession? When and why does a woman step beyond externally applied self-care and self-applied beauty products, to invasive procedures like Botox injections, lip plumping, face fillers and surgical procedures? And when does this spill over to become acute face and body image dysmorphia, a severe mental health condition that affects every age group and can lead to obsessive and excessive procedures?

Numerous studies have been undertaken to assess the effects on the general health and mental health of women who undergo enhancement and cosmetic surgery procedures, and how they feel afterwards. The results, in a nut-shell - some were delighted with the results whilst others were crushingly disappointed.

Those who were unhappy felt they didn't look how they thought they would look after the procedure. They had greater expectations and were now feeling dissatisfied and disappointed. This can often lead to further surgery requests, to keep trying for the exact look they wanted to achieve.

Studies into the psychological effects of those that undergo excessive cosmetic surgery procedures highlighted, that these patients are more likely to experience depression, social isolation, self-destructive behaviours and even suicide. It's a serious business from a mental health perspective, and that women are willing to get into considerable debt, often beyond their means, to pay for it.

Body image isn't always about cosmetic and surgical enhancements and trying to look and feel younger. Sometimes it's a weight-related health issue. Obesity continues to rise in the western world and bariatric surgery is not uncommon. These procedures are often the last resort for those who are obese and are suffering the associated risks and chronic health conditions.

It's all too easy to blame a person for their excessive weight, to point the finger and say it's their own fault - but it's far more complicated than that, and can cause immense misery for many of those affected. The weight loss industry has a lot to answer for.

THE WEIGHT GAME

How many of us have struggled with weight issues over the years? As you approach middle age it becomes very easy to gain weight and much harder to lose it. You'll be pleased to know that it's not entirely our fault - we can blame our fat hormones. We're going to meet these little buggers later.

Personally, I've had an erratic relationship with food most of my life. I was a skinny kid and young teenager. The teen magazines of the day had us believe that if you didn't look like Twiggy you were too fat, and I always thought I was fat.

I remember when I was about 13 and I asked my mum if I was fat. She said I looked like 'a drink of water dressed up' - meaning, if it wasn't for the clothes I had on, I would be invisible. I never believed her though and would periodically tell her I was going on a diet. She would just say okay and then make neck-end stew and dumplings for tea, because she knew there was nothing that would stop me getting my face into that!

From my early 20s I started to go through the weight-on-weight-off cycle. I continued to yo-yo diet through half of my life because I believed I needed to be a certain weight and if I wasn't, I was fat. There was no in-between. It was all about being a specific number on the scales. We believed all the weight loss gimmicks then, and the same hype is regularly regurgitated now. Each generation believes all the ideas are new and this latest one will definitely work, not realising it has been going around the block in numerous guises for decades.

Women who are now middle-aged, have lived through four, five or six decades of being told how to look, what to weigh, what to wear and how to wear it.

Bombarded in the early days with magazines and radio, then television, to where we are now - a massive overload and social saturation of media shit that tells us we're still not reaching the required standards!

And do you know why this hype keeps doing the rounds, decade after decade? It's because absolutely no-one can, or ever will, whether young, old or in-between, achieve the purported exacting standards of body weight, body height, body or face shape, for overall social acceptance. There's too much invested in it by the money hungry.

So many women feel they need to get on board with every 'new' diet that gets put out there, to try and stay ahead of the 'acceptable standard' game - one that has an ever-moving goal post. It won't ever be achieved, not whilst there's millions of dollars to be made in the beauty and weight loss industries, that make their fortune by creating, feeding and then pretending to resolve generations of female insecurities. I called time on it a long time ago and now I just see it for the bullshit that it is.

We can't leave the topic of body image without talking about the Body Positivity Movement, which started as a female solidarity rebuke to the beauty and weight-loss industries. The aim of the movement was to encourage, mainly larger women, to embrace who they are and accept how they look, and to stop focussing on negative body attributes. I remember when all this started and the focus was on overweight women, to accept themselves and to love their body and to push back the 'fat shamers'. This led to a flurry of larger ladies saying, "Fuck you haters, I love my big body", and parading around in skimpy underwear and tiny bikinis telling the world they were happy as they are and being big is not an issue for them.

Okay, that's great. I'm all for people accepting who they are and how they look and not giving a rat's arse what others think. What you look like and how you feel about it is your business.

Now here's the 'however'. If you are obese your body is struggling with an excess of fat, and how much fat you are carrying is an indicator of the number and level of health risks you face.

Being obese will dictate your level of mobility and ability to do everyday things.

But the far greater issue is the toll it's having on your body internally. There is visible fat and there's visceral fat, and it's the latter that can create a higher risk to your health and life expectancy.

Visceral fat is the fat that collects and settles around your internal organs bringing about a slow deterioration of your body's ability to function from within. It can prove fatal. The additional exertion your body requires for you to carry out your everyday movements is putting a strain on your heart and other vital organs. And that's just the beginning. This is not an exaggeration or fearmongering. It's fact.

Obesity is at epidemic proportions in the western world along with the associated health risks and health care costs. The biggest concern around obesity is not how you look, it's not even how you feel about how you look, and it's certainly not about what anyone else thinks about how you look.

Rationalising obesity and convincing women to be content with extremes of excess fat is not being kind, or understanding or supportive of feminist ideals, it's demeaning, patronising and dangerous. Ignoring the potentially life-threatening risks is not loving yourself.

Taking steps to reduce excess fat levels and potentially prolonging your life, is loving yourself.

I feel the initial intention of the Body Positivity Movement has been hijacked. It is inadvertently helping women to ignore the most important aspect of obesity - the detriment to their health and life-span - by feeding them a massive misdirection away from personal accountability and hiding it under a shroud of political correctness.

It's now considered offensive to describe someone as fat. Even if not used as a derogatory term. However, don't get bogged down with semantics. There is no necessity for anyone to get over-defensive about the word 'fat'.

As a certified weight-loss consultant and having coached many women on their weight-loss journey, I will say this - someone who exceeds their height/weight ratio and considered obese, is NOT 'fat'. They HAVE an excess of fat on and in their body. Fat is not WHO they are. It does not define them as a person. So yes, it is unacceptable to describe or refer to someone as 'fat' as though that is the only thing about them of any note or description.

As individuals we can look at ourselves and consider how well we function on a daily basis. We can decide ourselves if we are uncomfortable with our current weight and if it would be in our own best interest for our health to lose a few kilos. Now that we have reached middle age, let's stop pretending to be affronted, or jumping on the political and social bandwagons, and just accept it for what it is.

We've danced the dance many times in our decades of life. Just like when you were younger, whether you gain weight or not depends on what you eat, how much you eat, how active you are, genetics and any health problems you may have. But you can't use any of these as an excuse. Modifying your diet and your lifestyle to meet the changing needs of your body is and always will be, the key.

Practically all the things we go through during middle-age and menopause is linked to hormonal changes - but you can take control and lessen the impact.

Understanding your hormones and why we must do battle with them to maintain our health and our sense of self, makes the transitions easier to deal with.

Better the devil you know!

CHAPTER 4

HORMONE WARZONE

LET BATTLE COMMENCE

This is the part where we get down to specifics around what is happening to your midlife hormones. You can't avoid depleting hormone levels as you age, so if you are going to have to deal with all the crap that it brings, you might at least know why.

A woman is considered to have reached 'midlife' by the age of around 42. This is based on the current life expectancy of a woman which is 84. By age 42 your body has been working the previous 5 years or so for the changes to come. We are not considered 'old' until we are around 70-72 years. Good to know!

Now I'm not going to get all 'sciencey' or go into any great detail, but I do want to give you enough information so you can identify with it in relation to your own symptoms and experience as you head towards menopause.

I realise that some of you may already have reached menopause and are now into your 'beyond' years, but many of you will not be there just yet. Some will already know much of what I tell you here, some will know a few things and others will have a little or maybe, no knowledge. For this reason, we are going back to basics to meander through the effects of your changing hormones as you move through midlife, menopause and beyond.

During each phase of menopause your body is preparing you for what will be happening in the next phase. It knows exactly what it must do and will naturally just get on with the job. Hormones are team players, they don't work in isolation, so when a change occurs in one hormone, this has a knock-on effect on other hormones, and not usually in a good way. This causes biological and emotional turmoil that creates what I call the 'hormone-warzone'.

It is this battle that causes the symptoms we talk about as going 'through the change' or being 'menopausal'. Women can find this phase of their life to be difficult and debilitating.

The main hormonal changes occurring at this stage are to the female sex hormones oestrogen and progesterone.

Oestrogen is produced primarily in the ovaries and is responsible for the female reproductive organs and pregnancy. It is also responsible for all our female characteristics like our breasts and wider hips. Oestrogen affects bone health, brain function, elasticity of our skin, our sex-drive and our moods.

Sometime after the age of 35, the levels of these two hormones, that once ramped up to prepare you for pregnancy and motherhood, start to decline. Your body decides for you that you are beyond the optimum timeframe for becoming pregnant, because the likelihood of your body being able to support a healthy pregnancy is reduced. Your body responds accordingly making it more difficult for you to conceive.

As you move into your 40s, diminishing oestrogen levels trigger changes in your body and mental state. You may experience insomnia, sporadic irritability, stress and forgetfulness.

When oestrogen reaches a low enough level, you may start to experience the classic signs of perimenopause

- hot flushes, excess sweating at night, bladder issues and increased irritability. The tissues of the vagina and urinary tract may become dry. Sex may become uncomfortable or even painful and urinary-tract infections are common. It can also affect your bones, hair and blood vessels.

Progesterone is also produced in the ovaries, in the placenta and in the adrenal glands. When levels are balanced, it promotes sleep, anti-anxiety and feelings of being calm. It relaxes the smooth muscles of the intestines and other internal organs.

It also regulates the condition of your uterus and plays important roles in regulating the menstrual cycle and preparing your body for pregnancy.

But these two only play nice when balanced. As you age, and you enter the 'hormones gone wild' stage, it is predominantly oestrogen and its partner in mischief progesterone, who are to blame for the misery of perimenopausal symptoms throughout your 40s.

As age 50 looms on the horizon, declining progesterone levels affect the frequency of your menstrual cycle. Your periods will become irregular and may be heavier and more painful. Pre-menstrual migraines are common during this time, and you could find yourself feeling anxious or nervous and have heart palpitations. These are just a few of the most common symptoms and are part of the natural process of ageing and perimenopause.

An important reminder here is that it doesn't matter how light or irregular your periods are in the years up to menopause, it is still possible for you to become pregnant. Unless you want a baby very late in life, you will still need to take the necessary steps to avoid it.

Women also have testosterone. Although testosterone is considered a male sex hormone, women produce small amounts in their ovaries and adrenal glands. It is responsible for the growth and maintenance of female reproductive tissue and bone mass density.

Whilst oestrogen and progesterone are declining, other hormones are trying to adjust and compensate, but they too become unbalanced. This can lead to a whole host of other issues.

Not everyone has all the symptoms. Some women breeze through the phases of menopause with few symptoms, whereas others experience extreme debilitation. Although your declining hormone levels and resulting discomfort can affect your quality of life, they are not life-threatening.

If you think you may be perimenopausal but are not sure, ask your doctor to send you for blood tests. Don't be alarmed if you are told you are… those of us who have been through it survived!

Empowering yourself with knowledge is the key to your own good health and to successfully navigating the bumpy road ahead.

ROCKY ROAD TO MENOPAUSE
There is much you can do to alleviate the symptoms on the approach to menopause. Learning and understanding what you can do for yourself to help you through this phase of your life, will stand you in the best possible stead to advance healthfully through your 50s, 60s, 70s and 80s. Maybe even your 90s… who knows!

So, is menopause inevitable? For most women - yes.

Is it true that reaching middle age and experiencing menopausal symptoms can trigger feelings of uncertainty and pondering your purpose? For many women, it does.

Do you have to suffer through all these midlife changes in your body and mind as well as tolerate the often negative societal perceptions of 'the middle-aged woman'? Absolutely not.

One positive is that women no longer suffer in silence. Times have changed. It's not like in the 'old days' when women couldn't talk openly about menopause, menstruation or sex. These subjects were only ever mentioned in private, or in hushed tones - or not at all. They could never be spoken about in public and never ever in front of men! It would be considered quite indecent. People were embarrassed to say, hear or discuss such things.

Fortunately, women can now discuss menopause and their own symptoms quite openly. They can seek help and advice. Friend groups can sit in the pub and swap tales of hot flushes; joke about their forgetfulness; complain about being permanently pissed off with their varying levels of irritability; their lack of patience, sleepless nights and how really annoying they find absolutely everyone and everything all the bloody time.

Whilst perimenopause symptoms can be the subject of light-hearted banter, the associated impact can have a debilitating effect on a woman's day-to-day functionality, as she moves through the different phases.

The perimenopause phase can last between 1 and 10 years to around the age of 51. How you come through it can be largely managed by you. Learn all you can, how to eat and exercise, what are normal symptoms and what are not. Become better informed about hormonal changes so you know what to expect and how it may affect you.

Each phase of menopause can bring about many changes, not least the depletion of vitamins and minerals which causes aches and pains, poor digestion and a whole host of other symptoms that could be avoided if you have the right knowledge. The state of your health when you reach middle age and beyond, can be very much within your control.

The sneaky thing is that your focus during this time is on your menopausal symptoms and all the discomfort it is bringing. Then suddenly you realise what this means - you have reached middle age. It is from this revelation that women start to ask themselves questions about what they still want achieve and begin to contemplate life, the universe and everything, whilst simultaneously wondering how the hell middle age crept up on them with such stealth!

Menopausal age can be hereditary, and chances are you'll go through menopause at about the same age as your mother and grandmother did. There are other factors involved though. For example, women who smoke typically enter menopause two to three years earlier than those who don't.

Women who have had a hysterectomy and both ovaries removed, will experience symptoms of menopause straight after surgery, regardless of their age. For your body to work in harmony with itself, hormones need to balance. An imbalance can impact not just your physical health, but your mental health too - the way you think and the way you deal with problems.

Your self-talk can become negative and even generate feelings of hopelessness. Statistics show that the number of women who are diagnosed with depression doubles during her perimenopausal years.

How you look and feel when you reach midlife is greatly affected by the choices you've made and the life you have lived up to that point. There are of course other factors - like disease or illness - that could not be avoided and are totally out of your control.

Don't tempt fate. Make the decision not to wait and see what happens, if and how you will be affected and to what degree. Learn, read and ask questions... and then take the action required to put you in control. Your mind and body will thank you for it.

INCONCEIVABLE

Although reaching menopause is the end of a woman's journeys through puberty, pregnancy, motherhood and perimenopause, every one of us will have our own experiences along the way.

Many women don't know this - when a female baby is born, she will already have all the eggs she is ever going to have. As the years pass, the viability of those eggs will slowly decrease. After the age of 35, the rate of decrease becomes even more rapid, and a woman may find it harder to fall pregnant. I'm sure some of you will be able to relate to this.

Women who fall pregnant after the age of 35 are considered by the medical profession to be of Advance Maternal Age (AMA). A woman is most fertile from late teens to late 20s and professional opinion is that the best chance of a low-risk pregnancy and birth is between the ages of 25-29.

Although 35 is the age used as the marker for an older pregnancy, it is pregnancy in women over the age of 40 who are at most risk of complications for both the mother and baby.

I was an older first-time mum. I married for the first time when I was 25. Prior to getting married we'd talked about having children and he said he was on board with this. As one of seven children myself, I loved the idea of having a family of my own. However, early in the marriage when I brought up the subject that we should start thinking about a baby, he confessed that he didn't want any more children. He had two from his previous marriage and felt that was enough, even though their mother had remarried when both children were under seven, they lived overseas and he had no contact with them.

I felt bitterly hurt and disappointed that he was only just telling me this and I was crushed at the idea of never being a mother. Had I known he felt this way prior to the marriage it would likely have been a deal breaker. We stumbled through for 10 years but my feelings for him changed and dulled as the years went by.

The emotion of going through life childless was sometimes intense and I couldn't shake the feeling that he had purposefully deceived me. When the marriage eventually ended, I hoped in time I would find a new life partner who also wanted children, before it became too late for me to conceive. I was 35 - my eggs had already started 'going off', as someone indelicately informed me.

It was three years and four cats later that I met Ivan. We married two years after that, but it was established early on in our relationship that he was as keen as I was that we had a baby. We tried for 8 months to get pregnant to no avail. Because of my age we were referred early to a fertility clinic where I was jabbed and prodded and a myriad of tests were done.

Ivan's 'sample' had great swimmers we were told, and I had the fertility level of a 27-year-old. Despite my age, there was no evident reason why I couldn't have fallen pregnant naturally. I just didn't. I really wanted them to find something wrong so they could fix it. The closest we got to an answer was that, although my hormone levels were good, an imbalance in the perimenopausal mix was preventing my body from preparing for pregnancy. I was filed under the category of 'unexplained infertility'.

I was already 39 when we commenced fertility treatment. We underwent IUI (intrauterine insemination), and I fell pregnant. Three days before the 12-week milestone I suffered a 'missed' or 'silent' miscarriage. This is when the foetus stops developing or dies. The body doesn't recognise the pregnancy so does not expel the pregnancy tissue, meaning no miscarriage occurs.

The hospital wanted to wait to see if I would miscarry naturally. I didn't. I was left to carry my lifeless foetus for 3 days after which I was admitted to hospital for it to be taken away. The trauma of waking up on each of those mornings knowing I still had my 'baby' with me, but they were no longer alive, was indescribable.

We were told that the examination of the foetus showed they were severely Down-syndrome, and their heart had just not been strong enough to sustain life. We had been warned that this was a risk of a 'primigravida' pregnancy (when a woman is over 35 when she conceives) and suddenly it had become very real. I cannot even begin to describe the level of despair we went through.

We decided that we would try once more with IUI and if it didn't work, we would make a happy life with just the two of us. We knew we couldn't keep going through the emotional turmoil. I was so lucky to fall pregnant again. But at the 12-week stage, it looked like I would miscarry this baby too.

It was an anxious wait to see if the baby stabilised. She held on and started to thrive but at 32 weeks, my waters broke. The hospital tried to delay her birth for a couple of days, but she was having none of it. She was breech, feet down - clearly ready to hit the ground running, and it was decided she needed to be delivered by caesarean. I was scared at the prospect of giving birth almost 8-weeks early, but also happy and relieved. I just wanted her on the outside where I could see her.

I will never be able to adequately describe the feelings of love, relief and gratitude that were flowing out of me when she was safely delivered and I saw her tiny pink, scrunched up little face.

I was 41 years old when I gave birth to Rebecca. As an older first-time mum I was termed as 'elderly primigravida'. Basically, old, and pregnant for the first time. They could have called me a flying purple people eater for all I cared. I was just basking in the euphoria or knowing how lucky we were to have our baby and that I was at last, a mum.

The unflattering title of 'elderly primigravida' is bestowed on all women who become pregnant over the age of 35. We think at 35 we are still young, but for medical and reproductive purposes, we are not.

The lesson in this story is that hormones can be temperamental little shits, and you can't trust them. Your levels can be good but it only needs for something to tip the balance one way or another and a hormone war is declared.

To be fair, hormones are not really the villains of the piece. Whether we like it or not, hormones are the bringers of our pleasure and our pain, our rationality and our stability and when treated well, our good health. We need them, we must learn to love them and have a healthy and nurturing relationship with them. We can do this by understanding why they behave as they do, and how we can help them to function optimally - even when they're behaving badly and making us crabby.

MENOPAUSE – BRING THE CURTAIN DOWN

The word menopause is derived from the Greek words 'mens' which means month, and 'pausis' which means 'cessation of, or stop', and it marks the end of a woman's monthly menstrual cycle.

When you finally reach menopause it's a bit of a non-event. It occurs around the age of 51 and is marked by a woman realising that she has not had a period for 12 consecutive months. That's it. No fanfare, no brass band.

It seems an inadequate final bow for all the years of biological upheaval experienced on the approach to menopause. But on a deeper level, it is this single function that marks the permanent end to fertility and brings the curtain down on your reproductive years.

So that's it? Your periods have stopped and your childbearing years are over.

You've contributed to the world's population. Your purpose as a woman has been achieved. Thank you very much. You're done. Cheers!... So, what happens now?

The answer is... whatever the hell it is you want!

Middle-age and menopause just kind of creeps up and we become startlingly aware that we are more than half-way through life. But consider this, of the 40 years up to middle age, the first 18 years were dictated by others, until you became legally allowed to make decisions for yourself. That means only the latter 22 years were lived under your own control. You now potentially have another 40+ years for which you don't need anyone's permission to do whatever you want to do.

This time of your life should not engender feelings of getting old or being the beginning of the end, because it most certainly is not. It's another chapter of your life and you should embrace it with hope and enthusiasm, plans and goals. Think of it as an opportunity, a highlighted awareness. You can perceive it sadly that half your life is gone, or with joy at the prospect of a new beginning for the second half. This next phase can easily become the new, best years of your life. Travel this journey with a positive and open mind.

HORMONE REPLACEMENT THERAPY (HRT) – IS IT FOR YOU?

You will be aware that there are other solutions for menopausal symptoms, and it would be remiss of me not to talk about HRT (Hormone Replacement Therapy).

If you are really struggling with the symptoms of menopause, you can be prescribed HRT - which literally replaces the hormones depleted during the menopausal phases.

There are several forms of HRT. The main one is oestrogen replacement medication and another is progestogens, which is a natural and synthetic progesterone that can help with the sweating and hot flushes. Alternatively, your doctor may prescribe low-dose birth control pills to better control your erratic menstrual cycle.

It's important to remember that taking either birth control pills or HRT can make it more difficult to determine exactly when menopause has occurred, because your body is now being controlled by the drugs rather than going through the natural process.

There are some common side effects with HRT such as bloating, sore breasts, leg cramps, headaches and indigestion, but symptoms can be different for each woman. You may experience some, all, or none of these.

Be aware when you go to the doctor regarding menopausal symptoms that they will nearly always recommend and prescribe a pharmaceutical remedy rather than a nutrition and exercise remedy. Drugs as medicine is their role and their area of expertise - not nutrition.

You will find nutrition and exercise a highly beneficial remedy but if you go down a medicinal route, I hope that you don't make that decision lightly. You will need to discuss all the pros and cons with your doctor or other health care professional to consider if this is right for you.

Also remember that HRT is a short-term artificial solution whereas working on your diet, exercise and lifestyle can alleviate many menopausal symptoms in the early stages and set you up for great health for the rest of your life.

CHAPTER 5

BATTLE OF THE BULGE

You have now met and become acquainted with your sex hormones - and if you thought they were a mean and vindictive bunch, you are not going to be happy with the next group of hormones. After you have met these, it's likely you'll consider that your sex hormones are not so bad after all.

It was mentioned previously that the older you become, the more easily you gain weight - even though you haven't changed your lifestyle or your eating habits.

Well, here's the reason...

SAY HELLO TO YOUR FAT HORMONES!

If you are in the perimenopausal phase you may already be experiencing weight gain. To be fair, we can't wholly blame perimenopause and menopause for this. Although the phases of menopause are not directly responsible for causing weight gain, the symptoms created by hormonal fluctuations can make it harder for you to maintain and lose weight.

This is because hormones influence how your body uses and stores fat. They can affect your weight and energy levels and cause mood swings. As we go through this chapter you will start to see how the functions of some hormones cross-over and impact on one another. If there is an imbalance in one or more of your hormones, the effect and symptoms that result, can obstruct your efforts to eat healthily and lose weight.

Now I promised not to get too sciencey earlier, but it can be a bit difficult to simplify the convoluted process that is hormone behaviour.

You don't have to completely understand everything, there won't be a test… but you will get to understand that what you are experiencing is normal and manageable.

CORTISOL
You will likely have already heard of cortisol. It is known as the stress hormone, and it controls the release of glucose

(sugar). The higher your stress the more cortisol is released sending you to the cupboard for sugary snacks. Energy not used is stored in your fat cells.

Cortisol can help to control blood sugar levels and regulate your metabolism, the process through which your body burns energy (calories/kilojoules). It helps reduce inflammation and assists with memory formulation. Cortisol also has a controlling effect on salt and water balance in the body and helps control blood pressure. All these functions make cortisol a crucial hormone to protect your overall health and well-being. In middle age, as oestrogen and progesterone levels decrease, cortisol increases, and this contributes to weight gain.

INSULIN

The hormone insulin is responsible for keeping blood sugar levels within the normal range. It is made in your pancreas, and it allows glucose to move from your bloodstream into your cells to provide them with the energy to function optimally. It is known as the fat-storage controller. It regulates how the body uses and stores glucose and supports fat storage, meaning that any energy not used up by your cells is stored for future use. Insulin is a hormone that controls the metabolism as it breaks down the carbohydrates you eat and drink. This is why, when managing your weight, you need to keep a close eye on your intake of carbohydrates, which includes all starchy and sugary foods, and beverages.

GHRELIN

Ghrelin is the hormone released by your stomach to let your brain know that it's time to eat. For obvious reasons it is also known as the hunger hormone. But it has more roles than to just signal you are hungry.

This hormone also generates signals for the release of growth hormones. Low ghrelin levels can inhibit your hunger signals which doesn't sound so bad if you are trying to lose weight. However, low ghrelin can also trigger anxiety. And when we are anxious, cortisol is released, and where do we seek comfort - with food, particularly sugary and fatty foods.

Too high levels of ghrelin can increase your appetite and encourage you to eat more, so you need to keep your ghrelin levels balanced. Not just for the eating and weight factors, but because this hormone is also extremely important for heart health, bone metabolism and in preventing the breakdown of muscle.

LEPTIN

The hormone that regulates body weight is leptin. This is produced by your body's fat cells and is often referred to as the "satiety hormone" which basically means it signals your body to let it know that you are either full or still hungry.

Its main role is to regulate fat storage and how many units of energy you eat and burn, by turning on and off your 'I'm hungry' switch. If this isn't working as it should, the signal to stop eating is not received and leads to overeating. This can then lead to an excess of fat being stored resulting in you gaining weight.

SEROTONIN

Then there's serotonin, which is a natural mood stabiliser. Serotonin is a chemical that also acts as a hormone. It acts as a neurotransmitter that carries messages between the nerve cells in your brain and the rest of your body. Serotonin is known as the 'feel good' chemical as when it is at normal levels you are focused, calm and happy. As well as regulating your mood and social behaviour, it also impacts on your appetite and digestion, sleep, memory and even sexual desires.

When serotonin levels are low it creates a range of disorders, such as depression and anxiety, mood swings and mania.

It can become so bad that a person can have panic attacks and even suicidal thoughts. Low serotonin has been linked to post traumatic stress, obsessive behaviours and schizophrenia.

Too high serotonin levels can cause disturbed sleep patterns, poor digestion and bowel function and reduced bone density, making them weak and prone to fractures and osteoporosis. It is well documented that there is still so much more to learn about serotonin and its effects on the body, mind and disease.

THYROID

Last but not least is the thyroid. This little bundle of joy is a vital hormone gland that affects nearly everything.

Your thyroid releases two main hormones, T3 and T4, which together make up the thyroid hormone. It helps to regulate many of the body's functions by constantly releasing a steady amount of thyroid hormones into the bloodstream. The hormones released control your metabolism - that is, the way your body uses energy and burns fat. It also regulates your breathing and your heart rate.

An underactive thyroid means that the thyroid gland is not producing enough hormones. When this happens many of your bodily functions tend to slow down. You can have unexplained weight gain but also other symptoms that include tiredness, muscle weakness, heavier periods and feelings of depression. You may also experience irregular body temperature. Your cholesterol levels can be affected and may result in your arteries becoming clogged.

During health and weight-loss consultancy sessions, I had many women tell me they thought the reason they were overweight was because they have an underactive thyroid. It's possible, but not definitive. I would never assume this, and nor should you.

An over-active thyroid is when too much hormone is released causing increased metabolism and has the reverse effect of under-active thyroid. It results in weight-loss, an increased or irregular heart rate and increased hunger. You may find you are more tired and feel weak, sweat more and have problems sleeping.

Both underactive and overactive thyroid conditions can be debilitating and have serious health implications if left untreated

It probably did not escape your notice that many of the symptoms of both over and under active thyroid are similar to the symptoms of menopause. This is why it can be tricky if thyroid issues occur during the perimenopausal years. If you genuinely believe you have symptoms to suggest your thyroid is not functioning as it should, you should not ignore it. A number of diseases are associated with a malfunctioning thyroid such as hyper and hypo-thyroidism, Graves disease and Hashimoto's thyroiditis, and also thyroid cancer.

If you are experiencing ongoing symptoms, your doctor can refer you for blood tests and if necessary, prescribe medication or refer you to a relevant specialist. Dietary changes can help to manage symptoms but it's likely you will need some level of medical intervention.

BALANCING THE BEASTS

The overview of hormones given here barely scratches the surface of the importance of their role in every part of your physical and mental wellbeing.

Your hormones react to everything you do - when you eat, drink, socialise, what you do for a living, where you live and how you live your life. When you feel unhappy, lethargic or stressed, your body is sending you a message to treat it, and yourself more kindly. It's imperative you nourish and nurture your body and mind appropriately and treat them well. You will be rewarded by being able to lessen the negative effects of the natural process of middle age and menopause, and the years beyond.

Through diet to nourish, the replacement of lost nutrients to balance your hormones, exercise for bone and heart health, self-care, knowledge and understanding, you will know what you can do take to keep your hormones balanced. This will give you clarity and enable you to better control your day-to-day situations, thoughts and decision-making. This in turn will help to stabilise your moods, stress levels, weight and sleep patterns.

There is no magic formula, but by making a few well-placed adjustments to your everyday habits, you will feel massive benefits in all aspects of your life.

If you are already in the throes of menopausal symptoms it can be hard to get motivated to make changes when you already feel like crap. Although it may be more difficult to feel motivated, it doesn't mean you shouldn't make the effort.

When hormones are nurtured, balanced and working optimally, they will behave as nature intended, and you will feel good. However, when unbalanced, taming the beasts that unleash and cause all kinds of chaos will impact your capacity to deal and cope with everyday life events.

If you feel you have ongoing symptoms relating to anything that has been raised here, you should consider a trip to your doctor. A referral for simple blood tests can reveal the level of each of your hormones and identify a way forward in relation to mental wellbeing, better sleep, improved digestive issues and weight gain.

Midlife Weight Gain

An increase in weight, especially around your belly and mid-section is often associated with middle age. You can blame your hormones for many things, and although gaining weight is one of them, you shouldn't automatically assume they are wholly to blame and that you are completely absolved of any responsibility for your expanding midsection. There is always something you can do to take control of it before it starts to control you.

People are often described by the medical profession as either overweight or obese. It's important to understand that being overweight and being obese are not the same.

It's common for people to think being obese means someone is carrying much more weight than someone who is overweight. But it isn't. Overweight and obesity are not degrees of excess weight. They are degrees of excess fat. The terms 'overweight' and 'obese' refer to body weight that is greater than what is considered normal or healthy for a certain height. The issue is not, however, the number on the scales, but how much of that weight is fat.

Overweight generally relates to extra body fat AND may also be due to extra weight from muscle, bone or water. Being classified as overweight on ambiguous weight measure charts such as BMI does not automatically mean you are unhealthy or unfit, or even that you would benefit from losing some weight.

Obesity refers to those whose weight is excessively high due to the amount of excess fat they are carrying on their body and shows them to be well outside the healthy weight range for their height.

From middle age your muscle mass naturally starts to decrease, and your metabolism slows down. Muscles burn more energy than fat tissue therefore, as muscles decline, fat increases. Your thyroid controls your metabolism and your metabolic rate, which is the rate your body burns calories/kilojoules. Your metabolic rate is influenced by your age, gender, muscle-to-fat ratio and the amount of physical activity you do.

Between the ages of 20 and 60 your metabolic rate naturally slows down by around 22%. This means that your body is burning up calories at a slower rate over time, so as you age, you must eat less just to maintain the same weight.

At ages 40-50, you need to consume fewer calories every day than you did in your 20s and 30s, and by your 50-60s you need even less each day, just to maintain your weight. I know! It's not fair, it's bloody rude, but it's just the way it is.

On the plus side, knowing this means you can work with your changing body, readjust your eating quantities and/ or increase your activity levels.

Unless you have an underlying medical or physiological condition, your weight is mostly determined by how you balance your energy – the food and drink you consume everyday (intake) with the energy you use in your everyday activities (output). If you eat too much and exercise too little, the energy you don't use will be stored as fat. It's really that simple.

So many 'health gurus' want to overcomplicate this, and they have made it impossible to keep up with whatever the latest trend is. Do yourself a favour, stop lining the pockets of those who have got very rich by making you feel insecure and unloved and a failure for not being able to lose weight. They set you up for failure.

Start supporting your local grocer by buying unprocessed foods and making simple meals at home. I felt some eye-rolling going on there, but if you go back to basics, you will find it all much easier.

AND WHAT'S WITH THE BELLY FAT?

This one is a mega-frustration for many women. Unfortunately, the onset of belly fat is something that happens naturally in middle-aged women, especially after menopause. Your body fat tends to shift to the mid-section even if you're not gaining weight. This can be attributed to the decreasing level of oestrogen, which appears to influence where fat is distributed in the body.

As bad as you feel about how belly fat looks, you should be less concerned about this and more about what it signifies. I know it's important that we are satisfied with how we look, but there are some serious physical health risks that stem from having excess abdominal fat.

Belly fat can be subcutaneous fat, which is the extra layer of padding that sits just below the skin - this, on its own, is not a problem. However, a concentration of fat around your middle can also be an indication of visceral fat.

Visceral fat is not your friend. It lurks deep inside your abdomen, and gathers around your internal organs, your stomach, liver and intestines. Its equally unfriendly and unwanted sidekick is pericardial fat, which collects around your upper chest and heart.

Visceral fat is linked with serious health problems, including:

- Heart disease
- Type 2 diabetes
- High blood pressure
- Abnormal cholesterol levels
- Breathing problems

Again, not wishing to be alarmist, but research has associated belly fat with an increased risk of premature death (sorry, that *was* alarming) regardless of what a person's overall weight is. In fact, some studies have found that even when women were within a normal weight range, a concentration of belly fat increases the risk of cardiovascular disease.

So how do you know if you have too much belly fat? Let's be honest, we just know, don't we? Can't zip up your shorts, feel permanently bloated or even look pregnant. The simplest way to measure this is to measure around your waist. For women, a waist measurement of more than 80cm (35 inches) is a general indicator that you have an unhealthy concentration of belly fat and are at a greater risk of health problems.

Now those of you who know such things will no doubt recognise this as a BMI measure. But remember that BMI doesn't measure fat-to-muscle ratios. The increased risk of disease is triggered by the distribution of fat, specifically around the middle. If you had good muscle tone there, you'd likely have visible abs!

But here's the good news! Visceral fat is not indestructible. It responds to the same healthy diet and regular exercise strategies that help you shed excess kilos and lower your overall body fat.

What I say next I am sure you will have heard a gazillion times over the years. And there's a reason for it. It's what you need to do to be healthy. It's not a difficult concept and yet so many women want to make it difficult and dive into crappy weight loss trends (not judging - been there, done that).

The following points have always been the easiest, cheapest, healthiest, most effective, long-term solutions to weight loss:

- Eat a healthy diet
- Ditch sugary beverages
- Limit your alcohol intake
- Keep portion sizes in check
- Include physical activity in your daily routine.

Keeping within your healthy weight range is important. Weight gain in middle-aged women is seen as inevitable and even acceptable as 'just a sign of aging'. It isn't a foregone conclusion though, and it's a myth to suggest it's out of your control. Yes, it can be a natural part of ageing, especially if you have previously been active and are now leading a more sedentary life - but it doesn't mean you have to accept it. It is still within your control.

Losing weight can be more difficult when dealing with all the hormonal changes the phases of menopause bring. That said, don't convince yourself there is nothing you can do about it. For you to live a full and healthy life, you could start by not making excuses or absolving yourself of self-accountability.

If your hormones are misbehaving, maybe it's because you have not been engaging in enough self-care. That's not a criticism, it's a plea to you to start looking after yourself. If you want to be healthy and maintain a healthy weight you need to ditch the 'blame-game' mindset. Acknowledging that you might need to take some responsibility for your weight gain, because of your own unchecked habits, is a step towards acceptance. The sooner you can admit to yourself that you are the one who must make the changes, the sooner you can get on and do it.

Dump the idea of picking a weight and pushing yourself to achieve it. It is more likely to demotivate you than motivate. Instead, adopt a positive attitude and commit yourself. Write it down, say it out load, put notes up around the house stating – "I am going to lead a healthier lifestyle", "I will start eating healthier today", "I will incorporate exercise into my daily routine starting now". I know it sounds naff, but it can be effective and portends setting your intention and making a commitment to what you will do, how you will do it and when you will start - and serves as a reminder every day.

We have been conditioned to think that losing weight is difficult - and of course it can be - but it doesn't have to be. Your mind needs much more attention paid to it than your body does. If you don't believe in yourself, in your capacity to take control of the issue that is causing you to be overweight, be willing to make changes and accept that your current habits are harming you, you can't succeed.

If you keep making excuses and keep falling into the trap of quick fix solutions, there will be no long-term success.

How you think is how you feel is how you look and how you will be. Start believing in yourself and you are literally, 90% there.

CHAPTER 6

SURVIVING THE CONFLICT

LOOKING AFTER NUMBER ONE – NO IT'S NOT SELFISH
As the hormonal war for your body and emotions rage, there will be a need to choose your battles, put up your defences and make sure you are doing all you can to look after yourself. You can easily lose your sense of self, when old and new insecurities raise their ugly heads above the parapet. Nurture your self-worth, manage your self-esteem and look after your whole self. Being emotionally, nutritionally and physically fit will help you to come out of the other side without too many battle scars.

The importance of looking after yourself cannot be overpitched. As women, of course, most of us don't do it. It's been mentioned before, it is our nature to nurture and believe it is our role to make sure everyone else is okay before we bother to think about ourselves. Even when things are bad for us, we cover ourselves with a virtual band-aid and continue to nurture others. We might just want to curl up, shut out the world and tell everyone to fuck off. But we don't do that. Yes okay, maybe sometimes we do - we're only human.

Why is it so hard to prioritise ourselves? I believe we sometimes wear the 'martyr' hat. We ignore our own wants and needs and decide to take care of everyone else instead. It's a choice we make. We feel it's a requirement, an expectation, an obligation, call it what you will. When time is limited and let's face it, it always seems to be, we tend to other people's needs first and then there's no time for ourselves.

How often do you find that once you have finished tending to others, you feel irritable, frustrated, taken advantage of, resentful and tired. We nearly all feel this way, despite knowing we did it to ourselves.

If we do take time for us, or put our own needs before our partner, child or other family member, boss, colleague, clients - we feel selfish, even ashamed. We worry that other people will think we're being selfish - let's face it - we live in a pretty 'judgy' society.

But you can't keep putting that band-aid over everything and expect to stay functional, stress-free and happy.

Self-care is not selfish! It's not even just necessary, it's crucial to your health and wellbeing. So, engrain this into your psyche:

- You have to prioritise YOU!
- Prioritise your needs first.
- Looking after yourself is not selfish.
- The most important person in your life must be you.
- You cannot care for others if you don't care for yourself.
- Most people are not your responsibility.
- Other people's opinion of you is not your concern.
- Say 'NO' more often, especially if you feel someone is being unreasonable or taking advantage of you. Just say no.

Low Self-Worth or Low Self-Esteem

Some definitions of these have them interchangeable. Although they are related and have some cross-over with the emotional aspects, there are also subtle differences. Regardless, both can cause inner turmoil.

Put simply:

- Low self-worth relates to feeling like you are not worthy of love, affection and inclusion by others.
- Low self-esteem occurs when you rely on successes or achievements to define your worth.

Low self-esteem and low self-worth are something I lived with for many years, although at the time I either didn't know or didn't acknowledge what it was.

I left school at 16 with only one qualification, in English. I enrolled in a 2-year course at the local secretarial college but left after 6 months. I started Army life at 17, picking up the qualifications I needed to advance my career over the years, which I did successfully.

When I left the Army aged 31, I was back at what I considered at the time, to be the bottom of the heap. No real qualifications and no work experience outside of the military. It was unfortunate that the qualifications I had gained over the years were not linked to any recognition of prior learning certification outside of the military. Even though the work I had done had a totally transferable skillset, I had nothing to prove it.

I got a job as a civilian call centre operator for the local police. It was well paid, but I didn't enjoy it. I wasn't even good at it. I was a fish out of water and needed to get back to what I knew I was good at. I have always loved planning, organisation, writing, research and analysis - but didn't have the required qualifications to get my foot in the door to pursue this as a career.

One day I saw in the workplace weekly newsletter, details of Management and Public Policy courses being held at the local university. I decided that was it. That's what I needed to progress. I enrolled to do the part-time certificate over 12 months as I still needed to work full-time to support myself.

As the year of study was coming to an end, the head of the faculty spoke to me and offered me a place to stay on in a full-time capacity and complete the Honours Degree. I literally burst out laughing. I told him I would never be smart enough for that, people like me didn't go to university.

No one in my family had gone to university and I even feared my family would think I was "getting above myself" or had "ideas above my station" as the saying was. I thanked him for the offer, but I turned him down saying I couldn't do it.

He didn't say a word. He picked up a piece of paper and put a line down the middle. In one column he wrote the heading "Reasons to complete Degree Course" and on the other he wrote "Reasons I can't complete the Degree Course". He gave me the paper and told me to think about our conversation and write down my reasons under the relevant headings.

That night I dutifully wrote the two lists, so I could prove my point to him. I had about 10 reasons on the 'I can't do' side and 2 on the 'I should do' side.

The next day I gave the paper back to him. He read what I had written, tore the paper down the middle, screwed up the side that said, 'Can't do' and threw it in the bin. "Now we've got rid of your excuses," he said, "we can concentrate on why you should be doing this and get you enrolled". And that's what happened. His name was Don Pedrosa. I will never forget him.

His belief in me catapulted both my self-worth and self-esteem; I realised I had as much right to be there as anyone else. My new-found confidence and courage allowed me to pursue opportunities I would never have believed I was capable of.

I finished the degree with Honours, and I have never been more proud of anything in my life. But you know the funny thing? At the time, I wasn't doing the course so I could get a job that gave me more status or paid a bigger salary or even because I wanted to feel good about having gone to university. All of that came later as a happy consequence.

I had always felt embarrassed at my lack of academic qualifications. Part of me wanted to believe I could do so much more, but I was always shut down by another part of me that believed I was too stupid. I believed that if I could earn a degree it would prove I wasn't.

I later realised how irrational that was. Qualifications are proof of completing a course of education and acquiring a level of ability in learning. It is not proof of academic excellence, problem solving skills, common sense or capability.

Writing this reminded me of an occasion when my younger brother showed me I could be as dense as a bucket of sand. I was visiting my mum, it was about 35 years ago, and for reasons I can't remember, I wanted to store a television in her loft. I put a ladder up to the loft opening and mum and I were trying to figure out how to get the television up the ladder and into to the loft. The plan was that I would go into the loft, and she would pass the television up to me. It was never going to work. I was too short, Mum couldn't climb the ladder and certainly not holding a television that was heavy, and nor could I. It was too awkward to tie something around it to pull it up the ladder. We were still trying to figure it out a long time later when my brother came in. He asked what we were doing and when told, he said that he could do it by himself. I remember saying something snarky like – "because you're a man and you're bigger and stronger". He said "no, because I'm cleverer than you".

Mum and I laughed at his cockiness. Like me, my brother left high school with few qualifications, but he was smart, and he conclusively proved he was smarter than both of us. He went upstairs and came down with a sheet, he then went to the shed and got a length of rope. He tied the television up in the sheet, climbed up the ladder taking the end of the rope with him, got in the loft and winched the television through the gap. It took him about 5 minutes. It was so bloody obvious it was embarrassing and gave us all a good laugh. Common sense and problem-solving skills rolled into to one for a quick and successful outcome. Well played brother - well played – for proving once and for all that you don't need a university degree to outsmart someone who has one.

I came to realise that academic achievement wasn't, on its own, an indicator of intelligence, and that non-academic skill sets - problem-solving, leadership qualities, emotional and social intelligence and creativity, are just as valid.

I believe my neurosis manifested from being told by a teacher in middle school that I was stupid, because I couldn't grasp some mathematical concepts. My brain just wasn't wired that way. After he yelled at me and called me stupid in front of the whole class, I think I mentally checked out. I learned nothing more in maths, mainly because I stopped going to his lessons. I still remember his name - but I won't put it here in case the nasty, miserable bastard is still alive.

All that aside, the insecurities I felt around this disappeared when I walked up on to the stage and was awarded my degree. I was no longer the person without any qualifications. I no longer cared if people thought I was stupid and uneducated. I no longer cared one jot about other people's opinion of me, in that regard. On the other hand, nor did I feel that because I had a degree, I must now be intelligent - I just felt that maybe I hadn't been as stupid as I'd believed I was.

Let me say again here, my feelings about lack of qualifications were my hang-up, my insecurity, my rock-bottom self-worth and self-esteem issue. I think I might be worried I'm projecting my insecurities here!

That said, the achievement was the turning point for me on so many levels because along with it, my self-worth grew immensely. Prior to making the decision to go full-time at university I was going through a divorce, having walked away from 10 years of marriage with absolutely nothing but my personal belongings. It was emotionally draining on so many levels, but the right decision.

Prior to my decision to continue the course I had just signed the mortgage on a little terraced house and taken out a hire purchase agreement on a second-hand car (two of the reasons on my 'I can't do the course full time' list along with 'I need to work to pay for them!'). To this end I continued to work almost full-time hours, in the evenings and at weekends; money was still really tight and I felt permanently knackered!

All the younger students (I was twice their age, they called me Mum!) had fancy computers, but I only had an old-fashioned Word Processor to complete my assignments on. My saving grace was that I was now totally committed to completing the course. I knew I was going to keep going no matter how hard it was. I found strength and resilience within me I didn't know I was capable of, and I believed in the power of determination and commitment. With that, and a large serving of sheer bloody-mindedness, I got through it.

I believe all the difficulties, and coming through them, contributed to bringing me all the good things that followed. It was me believing in myself. The thing I am most proud about is the person I became going through what were at that time, the toughest years of my life.

I haven't always liked myself, but I am not embarrassed to say I like myself now. I am proud of what I have achieved. I like who I became through adversity, and I love the life I have created.

I'm sure many of you have similar stories of hardship that you have overcome through resilience and resolve, to achieve many things you are proud of. It doesn't matter how big or small the obstacle you got over was. You conquered it. You proved to yourself you could, and you did. No one else's opinion matters. Don't be afraid to congratulate yourself and feel bloody good about it.

BE PROUD OF WHO YOU ARE
It's a sad fact that, like I once did, too many women play down their role in life because they fear they will be judged.

When you meet people for the first time and they ask you about yourself, and what you do for a living - how many of you say "oh, I'm just"… this, or just that as though what your role is, at that time in your life, defines you as the woman you were, are now, or will become.

You are not a lesser or greater person than anyone else because of what you do for a living. You are not defined by your job. Your role in society is important, no matter what you do, whether you're a doctor or you work in a supermarket. You are fulfilling a role in the community and contributing in different ways. If it wasn't for their workforce, a CEO of a company would not have a business or a job. Many of them would do well to remember that.

You are not 'just' a housewife, you don't 'just' work as a secretary, you are not 'only' a cleaner or an admin assistant. You are not 'just' or 'only' anything. Whatever it is you do, don't demean it or yourself by playing it down. You are earning a living; you are supporting yourself and maybe others. What you do for your job has a purpose and you have a goal.

If you decide you want to pursue something else, there's nothing to stop you from exploring the possibilities and creating other opportunities. But do it for yourself. You have the power to totally control your own narrative without needing to talk yourself up or put yourself down.

Continue to challenge yourself whilst setting realistic goals, to nurture yourself and to grow, be proud of your achievements and most of all, be kind to yourself,

The saying "You only get one chance to make a first impression" is very true. You should always be your authentic self. If people don't like or accept you, that's on them. They are not your people.

CHAPTER 7

LET'S TALK NUTRITION

BACK TO BASICS

It's time to change tack and move from matters of mental conditioning to physical and nutritional habituation - although all are interconnected.

The importance of good nutrition has been mentioned throughout previous chapters, but now we are going to get down to specifics. If you have been pondering your state of health and what you can do to improve it, a good place to start is with an overhaul of your eating habits. Living healthfully can be as simple and inexpensive as it has always been. Or it can be as difficult and expensive as you make it.

You may already feel that you eat and exercise well, but what worked for you in your younger years may not still be working for you now. You may not even have noticed the subtle, and not-so-subtle clues your body has been sending you.

Each of you will have different levels of knowledge and understanding of what good nutrition is. To make sure everyone leaves this chapter with a better understanding of how best to fuel your body, we are going back to basics. If you already know a lot, great, this will be a refresher. If you don't, no problem, you will benefit from what you learn here.

WHY DO WE EAT?

I asked this question in a group client meeting once and someone said, "so we don't die". Well, yes, that's basically it. But it's more about supplying the body with what it needs for you to stay alive <u>and</u> remain healthy.

Food provides the body with the essential nutrients it needs so you can live a long, healthy, functional and independent life. You can get the range of nutrients you need by consuming a wide variety of foods from across the different food groups. So it's not just about eating food, it's about eating the right food, in the right amounts, for nutritional balance and weight management. It all sounds so simple. And, theoretically, it is.

Unfortunately, living healthily was hijacked many years ago by the big weight-loss, beauty and pharmaceutical industries and turned into a multi-million-dollar industry that saw money to be made from the insecurities of others. In promising much and delivering little, we are led to believe that we need to fork out lots of cash for pills, potions, shakes and whatever wonder drug is trending, to be healthy and lose weight. By jumping on this bandwagon, the only thing guaranteed to be lighter is your bank account.

The vast majority are crank schemes aimed at reeling you in with fantastical claims. They just want your money! Don't think I'm saying this and implying I have never fallen for it. I have, many times over the years.

Living healthy is a state of mind. It can cost you no more than your commitment and determination to not take the short cuts, which will only leave you disappointed and disillusioned and without long-term results.

If you decide that living healthily as you age is something you want to achieve, you will need to be open to making the required lifestyle changes. It requires commitment to yourself to do what needs to be done, to take control of your thought processes and train your mind and body to work together for the benefits it will bring. Whether you want to change to healthier eating for your overall health or for weight loss too, it's achievable. But the only person who can do it, is you.

I'm not going to go into detail regarding the biochemical and physiological processes of how the body uses food because it can get heavy and feel overwhelming. I don't want you to put it into the 'too hard' basket before you even start. Instead, an overview of the basics will put you in the right frame of mind to get you thinking - without over-thinking!

MACRONUTRIENTS

Carbohydrates, protein and fat are collectively known as macronutrients. Within each of these food groups there is a further breakdown but basically, everything you consume is classified under these food groups. Different food items have different nutrients required by your body for specific functions. This is why it's crucial to eat a balanced variety of food from each group.

Most of you will have first learned the information I am about to give you in school biology lessons. But that was a long time ago, so we're going to revisit and refresh your memory.

CARBOHYDRATES

There are two general types of carbohydrate: simple and complex. Simple carbohydrates are sugars. These are the quickest source of energy, as they are rapidly digested. Unfortunately, most foods high in simple carbohydrates contain few nutrients and high kilojoules/calories. They also lack fibre so pass into the bloodstream quickly which creates a feeling of needing more food, leading to over-eating.

Some examples of simple carbohydrates:

- White/brown sugar
- Corn syrup
- Honey
- Maple syrup
- Jams, jellies
- Fruit cordial
- Soft drinks

Complex carbohydrates digest slowly, so they keep blood sugar more stable than simple carbohydrates do. They are often rich in fibre, more satisfying, and more health promoting.

Complex carbohydrates are commonly found in whole plant foods and generally high in vitamins and minerals.

These whole plant foods are great sources of complex carbohydrates:

- Green vegetables
- Fruit – that is high in fibre. (Fruit contains both simple and complex sugars but either way, fruit is generally good for you.
- Whole grains, such as oatmeal, pasta, brown rice and wholegrain breads
- Starchy vegetables - potatoes, sweet potatoes, corn, and pumpkin
- Legumes – Kidney and black beans, chickpeas, lentils and peas

MACRONUTRIENT - PROTEIN

Protein is an essential part of a healthy diet and no, it doesn't need to be in the form of meat. Proteins are the nutrients that are building blocks called amino acids. Your body uses amino acids to build and repair muscles and bones and to make hormones and enzymes.

Protein is the basis of the structure of hair and skin. It can also be used as an energy source. There are so many sources of protein both animal and plant-based so make sure you have a variety.

Include:

- Meat (sparingly)
- Poultry
- Eggs
- Fish
- Nuts
- Seeds
- Legumes and beans
- Tofu, soybeans and other soy products

MACRONUTRIENT - FAT

Fats are the nutrients in food that the body uses to build cell membranes, nerve tissue (including the brain) and hormones. The body also uses fat as fuel. If fats eaten aren't burned as energy or used as building blocks, they're stored by the body in fat cells.

A small amount of fat is an essential part of a healthy, balanced diet. Fat is a source of essential fatty acids, which the body cannot make itself, and it helps the body to absorb vitamin A, vitamin D and vitamin E. These vitamins are fat-soluble, which means they can only be absorbed with the help of fats.

Healthy fats include:

- Olive oil
- Avocado
- Nuts
- Fish that is high in Omega 3s - Salmon

Fat helps give your body energy. It helps to protect your organs and supports cell growth. It has a role in keeping cholesterol and blood pressure under control, and helps your body absorb vital nutrients. Many people see fat as the enemy but if you cut fat out of your diet, you will be depriving your body of what it needs to function healthily.

Like most things in life, the food in each of these food groups is not created equal. That is, there are good and not so good carbohydrates and it's the same for protein and fats. Learning which benefit you, and which hinder your health and weight loss efforts, will stand you in good stead in controlling your weight and maintaining good health.

MICRONUTRIENTS – VITAMINS & MINERALS

Vitamins are organic substances, which means they derive from living matter, and they are either fat soluble or water soluble. Our bodies are unable to produce them, and we must get them from the food we eat.

Minerals are present in soil, water and rocks. They are inorganic and are absorbed into plants. Animals eat the plants and we eat both plants and animals.

You will likely be aware of magnesium, zinc and copper, but there are many other minerals you may not be so familiar with that your body needs in only trace amounts. To maintain health and hormonal balance, support your immune system and maintain a healthy heart and bones, it is essential you get them in the food you eat.

The only way you can get all the vitamins and minerals your body needs is to eat a wide range of food from each of the food groups and sub-groups. You can buy food that is fortified with vitamin and minerals but be careful of this. Many of these are packaged and processed foods that may not be healthy in other areas and will have added preservatives to extend their shelf-life.

Alternatively, if you are not getting all the vitamins and minerals you need from your food, because of specific dietary requirements, you could take supplements.

However, it's not recommended that you take supplements unless you have been diagnosed as deficient by a health professional. It can be confirmed by a simple blood test, and depending on the levels, supplementation may be advised. That said, you would be better advised to increase the foods you eat that contain your deficient vitamins and minerals. Taking supplements when you don't have a confirmed deficiency can upset the balance within your body and cause you any number of digestive issues and hormonal imbalances.

WATER, WATER EVERYWHERE

You need to drink water! Yes, I know you've heard this ad nauseum, but there's good reason - your body needs it to function!

The average female's body is made up of about 55% water. Here are just a few examples of the role water plays in our well-being:

- It is the primary building block of cells.
- It metabolises protein and carbohydrates in food.
- It regulates body temperature.
- It is the main component of saliva which aids food breakdown and digestion.
- It carries oxygen and nutrients to cells.
- It flushes out toxins when we pee!

Drinking water is such a simple thing and yet so many of us find it hard to do. Try and make it a habit that you always have access to water. If you go out and don't know if water will be available, take a bottle with you.

SUGAR

When people think of the impact of too much sugar they generally think of excess weight. But that isn't all. Excess sugar can also:

- Trigger type 2 diabetes
- Supress your immune system
- Inhibit the absorption of key minerals
- Bring on mood swings
- Reduce collagen and elastin in the skin… causing wrinkles!
- Cause you to gain weight.

Sugar is addictive. It triggers good feelings in the brain, and a lack of it can bring on withdrawal symptoms that will cause you to seek out more of it. The good news is that you can be break your addiction to sugar and improve your health.

Get into the habit of checking food labels. So many products contain 'hidden' sugar. Sugar has many identities, and if you see the following words on a label - fructose, lactose, glucose, dextrose - it means sugar. Basically the '...ose' signifies a type of sugar. Watch your drinks too, they can have a crazy amount of sugar in there without you even knowing it.

EXERCISE & FITNESS

Don't tell yourself you don't have time to exercise. You know it's not true. You will never find the time to do something you don't really want to do. You must prioritise it and value its importance to your overall health and wellbeing.

It doesn't matter how old you are or what medical condition, injury, joint or mobility issues you have, it would be extremely rare that you would be advised by a health professional not to take part in any form of physical exercise, activity or exertion. Any extension of incidental movement is beneficial.

Continuing some form of exercise is essential for your heart, muscles, bones, mental health and weight management.

If you already exercise regularly that's awesome. If not, how can you get into the habit of daily exercise? The easiest way is to find an exercise you really like and prioritise it, factor it into your day - not just say "I'll do it if I have time". Make time. Make yourself accountable.

I'm currently waiting for knee replacement surgery. My orthopaedic consultant warned me there are activities I should no longer do. Like, he thought it was a bad idea that I periodically climb the pear tree in our garden with my chainsaw to lop off the top branches.

It's frustrating not being able to do this, I found it therapeutic. Especially after a day that had too many people in it. The symbolism of lopping branches off a tree with a chainsaw is far more satisfying than sticking needles into a voodoo doll. I digress. I will dutifully heed his warning - no more tree climbing. For now.

He did tell me the kind of activities I could still do to stay active and mobile before and after my surgery though. I shall be a good patient and do only what he has recommended because I want to get back into everything as soon as possible.

Movement is essential to help with healing, flexibility, muscular and bone strength. The key is to find something you enjoy, within your limitations - and then do it regularly. You will feel more energised, clear headed and focussed.

It will release stress and tension, help to control your weight and regulate your sleep pattern. There are no 'get-out' clauses and no excuses.

Chapter 8

Heart, Bones, Digestive & Respiratory Health

In previous chapters I've mentioned a variety of health measures relating to healthy heart, bones and digestion. I am also including respiratory health here. We are going to get into some specifics, and double-down on your understanding so that you know what actions you can take to combat known risks in women after the age of 40.

Bone Health

Bone health is a massive issue as women age. It's the deterioration of bones that bring about the end of an active life for many women which can lead to the onset of other issues, such as joint stiffness and weight-gain.

Your skeleton undergoes a natural process throughout your life of constant break down and regeneration of the underlying structure of collagen and minerals. This is what keeps your bones strong. You don't just get to a certain age and suddenly have weak bones, but your bone mass will have reached its peak around the age of 30 and will remain constant for around 15-20 years.

The breakdown-regeneration cycle slows down when deprived of nutrients, and women over the age of 50, especially after menopause, have the greatest risk of developing osteoporosis. When the bone renewal process can't keep up with the breakdown of old bone tissue, it causes bones to become weak and brittle - so brittle that a fall or even mild stresses such as bending over or coughing can cause a fracture. Osteoporosis related fractures most commonly occur in the hip, wrist or spine.

There are several factors that can increase the likelihood that you will develop osteoporosis. Some factors are within your control, for example your lifestyle choices, such as whether you smoke or drink an excess of alcohol, but there are other factors that fall outside of your control.

Ageing in general can prompt your body to leach calcium from your bones. Over time, your body becomes less efficient in absorbing calcium and other nutrients needed to maintain a healthy level of bone density. Being a woman means you are four times more likely to develop osteoporosis than a man, and the older you get, the greater your risk. If you have a family history with a parent or sibling having osteoporosis, this also puts you in the higher risk bracket.

Small women tend to be at a higher risk. Their body frame size means they will have less bone mass to draw on as they age. If your ethnic origin is white or Asian, you too will be at greater risk of developing osteoporosis. And those with certain medical conditions, resulting treatments and prescribed medications, can all contribute to and exacerbate the natural age-related decline of bone mass.

But don't put this into the 'too hard' basket. Your willingness to feed your bones the right nutrition and to undertake regular weight-bearing exercises is vital for bone health and for keeping active as long as possible. This is an occasion where a supplementation may be recommended.

MUSCLE HEALTH

From as early as your late thirties you will naturally start to lose muscle mass. This too is a normal part of ageing and is called sarcopenia. There are hormone receptors in our muscles, and during perimenopause, this brings about further decline of muscle mass as hormone levels drop.

Typically, a woman will lose about 3-5% of muscle mass every decade and this rate can accelerate to around 8% after the age of 40. It can then almost double after the age of 70. A natural mechanical process is for muscle and bone tissue to work together and interact. When both are in decline you will notice that your strength and power to hold and grip will also decrease.

The loss of muscle affects not just strength, but balance, and can lead to an increased risk of falls and fractures. And because menopause also contributes to a decline in muscle strength, this is a crucial factor in the decline of functional independence in old age.

That said, initial signs of frailty can begin as early as in your 30s and 40s, so don't wait until you start showing physical signs. Building up bone and muscle resilience in your younger years is really important. It can save you from losing your independence in later life because you no longer have the strength, flexibility or energy to do things for yourself.

At the risk of sounding like a broken record, the way to do this is to have a healthy relationship with our old friends, 'Good Nutrition' and 'Regular Exercise'. Good nutrition, maintaining a balanced diet, and being active are ways to support your muscle health that is totally within your control.

Just like you need oxygen to breathe, you need to nourish your muscles with protein and Vitamin D, to combat the breakdown of muscle.

THE HEART OF THE MATTER

Just because you are ageing, it doesn't mean you have to give up looking after yourself. The sooner in your life you start making changes, the longer you will feel the impact for all the years in your future.

Making healthy choices during any decade of life increases the chances of staying healthy as you age. It is increasingly reported by health professionals that, regardless of your age now, whether it's 35 or 75, you can take control of your health and greatly reduce your risk of heart disease, now and in the future.

The Heart Foundation identifies factors that will help you to lower your risk of heart disease:

- Maintain a healthy weight.
- Eat more fruits, vegetables and whole grains.
- Quit smoking.
- Modify alcohol consumption.
- Regular exercise, even if it's just a walk around the block.
- Eat varied and nutritionally balanced meals.
- Improve cholesterol levels.
- Lower blood pressure.
- Control diabetes.
- Learn to manage stress.
- See your doctor for regular checkups to monitor your heart health.

You may during your perimenopausal phase notice your heart skipping a beat. You may also experience the beat of your heart appearing slower or the opposite, experiencing palpitations - an increase or fluttering in your heart rhythms. The reason for this, once again, is that troublemaker oestrogen - or should I say lack of oestrogen.

The role of oestrogen in the heart is to keep your arteries flexible. During the menopausal phases, you can have significant fluctuations of oestrogen production. These fluctuations cause your arteries to dilate or contract.

Oestrogen has a protective influence on the heart, but its effect becomes compromised, which can create a higher risk of cardiovascular problems, including an increase in the risk of high blood pressure and hypertension.

As soon as you cross the threshold into your 40s, the many changes that start to take place in your body can increase your risk for developing heart disease. That said, the phases of menopause don't cause cardiovascular disease, but higher risk factors can begin to occur around this period of a woman's life.

Women aged 40 to 59 represent 5.6 percent of all the people who have heart disease. This may not sound too extreme until you consider that the risk is less than 1 percent for women up to their 30s.

The natural wear and tear of living many years of life will affect your health - even if you have been mindful about managing other risk factors. As you age, changes in the structure of your blood vessels naturally occur. You'll find that during physical activities your heart beats faster than it once did for the same exertion.

As time goes on, your heartbeat can become irregular resulting in a gradual thickening of the heart walls. These changes are a normal part of ageing, but they can increase your risk of heart disease and heart attack.

If you have concerns about any symptoms you are experiencing, you should never ignore them and consult your healthcare professional without delay, for advice and a check-up.

Cholesterol

There are two types of cholesterol. For simplicity, there is good cholesterol (HDL) and bad cholesterol (LDL). You may be familiar with the associated risks of cholesterol imbalance, that can trigger heart disease. Young people can be diagnosed with high cholesterol, but it is most commonly diagnosed in people between ages 40 and 59. This is because, as you get older your body's metabolism changes, and your liver is not able to remove the bad LDL cholesterol as well as it did when you were younger. Although these are normal changes, it may increase your risk for developing increased blood cholesterol levels as you age.

Blood Pressure

Healthy blood pressure readings should be close to 120 (systolic) over 80 (diastolic). Next time you get your blood pressure taken, ask your doctor what your reading is and if it is higher or lower, what does this means for you.

If your blood pressure is significantly high, it can cause the heart muscle to thicken. This increases the amount of work your heart has to do and may lead to heart disease or even a heart attack. Listen to your body and be aware of any changes to your heart rate or other symptoms like dizziness or blurred vision. No doubt your doctor will let you know if there is any cause for concern.

Respiratory Health

Smoking is the number one cause of respiratory disease in women. Those of you who smoke, please swallow your urge to get defensive. Yes, it is your choice, and you can accept or discard the information if you wish, but the facts and possible consequences remain true.

Cigarette smoke contains over 7,000 chemicals. Tobacco is the biggest cause of cancer in the world and smoking is known to be the direct cause of at least 16 types of cancer. It is the primary cause of emphysema and exacerbates other debilitating respiratory conditions such as bronchitis, asthma and chronic obstructive pulmonary disease (COPD), all of which could seriously impair the quality of your life and lead to an early death. Alarmist? It is what it is.

Most people know, smokers and non-smokers alike, that smoking is likely to cause some level of disease in your body. It may or may not be life-threatening for you, but even if you live to a good age, the quality of your health and life will diminish with each year you continue to smoke.

I often hear, when talking to clients, family and friends who smoke, that they acknowledge they could contract a smoking-related disease or die of cancer but believe they could just as likely get hit by a bus and die anyway. Sigh.

Well yes of course they could, but that would be an unfortunate accident. You wouldn't test the theory of being maimed or killed by deliberately stepping out in front of a bus. That would be bloody stupid. But smoking is a conscious and deliberate act that people do, many times a day, every day, every week for countless years. I can't help but wonder why anyone would want to play Russian roulette with their life. As judgmental as this sounds, it really is a genuine, "Why the fuck would you do that?"

My dear Gran, whom I loved dearly, was a heavy smoker who lived until she was 84. However, the quality of her life for the last 25 years was seriously debilitated. Her breathing was laboured, and you could hear it making crackling noises. You could hear her wheezing from the next room. I was with her when she died of lung cancer, delirious from the pain medication but still groaning and calling out in pain.

Lung cancer is a horrible disease that also took both of my parents, both heavy smokers. My dad was only 52. My mum was 70. Both were too young to die. I was at the hospital with my mum when she was diagnosed and told she had late-stage lung cancer, that would take her life in 6-9 months. She told me that she didn't want to die and asked me if it would help if she stopped smoking straight away. The pain in my heart at hearing her ask that was unbearable. All I could think was, if only she had considered that many years sooner. She died 10 months later. My heart broke.

I am not denigrating the smokers amongst you, as I said, I don't understand it but accept it is totally your choice, and I'm sure you are fully aware of the risks. It's also unlikely you are not aware, that it would be better for your health and pocket if you stopped. If you do want to quit, there are plenty of support mechanisms around to help you, via your doctor, pharmacy or even hypnosis.

DIGESTIVE HEALTH

Not enough importance is attached to the digestive system, which is the source of all health. In recent years there has been much research, written and substantiated regarding the correlation between your brain and your gut. The brain-gut connection highlights the links between thought processes, digestion, mood and many aspects of health.

The digestive system has a role in so many bodily functions. It's where you get nutrition to feed every cell in your body and support for your immune system. If it is inflamed or you are constipated, you will feel uncomfortable and irritated. The knock-on effect of your discomfort can bring about other ailments, including anxiety and other mental health conditions. When your digestive system is not functioning optimally, it can't do its job, and your health will decline as a result.

As our age number gets higher, our body lets us know, sometimes indelicately, that things are not functioning as well as they used to. More than half of all women report frequent gas, diarrhoea, constipation or painful bloating. These are signs of poor digestive function and can lead to an inability to absorb nutrients for efficient distribution throughout the body. This can lead to a whole host of problems for older women for a number of reasons:

- Our hormones have changed but we don't modify our food intake as we age.
- We continue to eat the same food in the same amounts as we have previously, but our digestive

system can no longer cope with it the way it used to.

- We produce less saliva.
- We don't move as much as we should.

With declining hormone levels comes a decline in vitamins, minerals and enzymes. These deficiencies can cause intolerances that you may not have previously had, like becoming lactose or gluten intolerant.

Gluten, dairy, and other food intolerances can adversely affect your gut microbiome, the healthy bacteria in your gut. This paves the way for leaky gut, chronic inflammation, and potential autoimmune disorders. Looking after your gut can fix many problems you hadn't even realised you had and were related.

These are ways you can help your digestion:

- Chew your food longer.
- Keep hydrated.
- Eat smaller meals.
- Exercise regularly, even if it's just walking.
- Maintain a healthy weight.
- Check with your doctor for vitamin/mineral deficiencies or any newly acquired food intolerances.

Where possible you should always get your nutrients, vitamins and minerals from your food. However, it's unrealistic to think that this is always possible, especially as you get older. Even though you may have a wide and varied healthy diet, your body cannot absorb and distribute the nutrients as efficiently as it did when you were younger.

The key is to be more mindful of the signals your body is giving you and make changes to your eating habits. If this doesn't help, seek professional advice.

You will need to eat less just to maintain your weight and even less again if you want to lose it. We can all say that we don't feel any different than we did years ago. Whether you accept it or not, your body is different, your hormones are changing, your metabolism is slowing down and your food intolerances are going up. For all these reasons you need to be more mindful of what you eat and drink and make better choices.

LIFESTYLE FACTORS

Excess alcohol use, cigarette smoking, poor eating habits and lack of exercise can all increase your risk of heart disease.

Smoking reduces the flow of blood to the heart and speeds up the clogging and narrowing of the coronary arteries which can lead to a heart attack.

Alcohol is a major risk factor for heart disease and directly impacts other risk factors such as your blood pressure/ hypertension. High blood pressure causes your blood to be pumped more forcefully through your arteries, which can lead to a stroke or heart attack.

Type 2 diabetes is caused when the body is unable to make sufficient levels of the hormone insulin or, the insulin that is released is not working as it should. Despite there being genetic links, type 2 diabetes may be preventable. Poor diet and other lifestyle habits are considered the bigger factor in a significantly high number of type 2 diabetes cases.

Insufficient insulin will cause the level of glucose (sugar) in your blood to become too high. Increased factors are:

- Age – especially after the age of 45.
- Fat distribution – particularly relating to visceral fat around internal organs.
- High cholesterol – plaque (fatty build-up) in blood vessels affect regulation of blood sugar levels.

- Poor diet – high in fat and sugar, will cause weight increase and excess fat.
- Inactivity – lack of exercise.
- Smoking – damages cells making the body less responsive to insulin.

Once you have type 2 diabetes there is no cure. However, you can put it into remission by losing weight, changing to a healthy diet and exercising regularly, therefore negating the need for life-long medication.

ACTIVITY LEVEL

Research has shown that exercising regularly in middle age can improve the elasticity of blood vessels brought on by a sedentary lifestyle and reduce cardiovascular disease risk.

The best kind of exercise in middle age and beyond is core training, free weights training and cardio. Engaging in these three types of exercises will benefit the health of your heart, bones and muscles.

Lack of regular exercise, especially after the age of 40, puts you at greater risk of heart problems. Regardless of how busy you think you are, it's important to find time for moderate to vigorous physical activity, such as walking or swimming on a regular basis. Regular exercise also helps to control other risk factors, for example blood pressure and cholesterol.

You may not be able to run a marathon, nor is it necessary to strive for this. But regardless of your current fitness and mobility levels, there will always be something you can do. No matter how little that is, it will always be more beneficial than doing nothing at all.

STRESS

We live in a fast-paced society and many of us go through periods of stress. Others live with long-term chronic stress. Stress causes the hormone cortisol to increase, which can increase blood pressure. The release of adrenaline during stressful situations can cause the heart to beat faster and in turn increase blood pressure.

Stress is an unseen condition that can be totally debilitating and bring about an increased risk of a heart attack or stroke. Reducing stress in your life is an absolute must and an essential factor in living healthily.

EXISTING HEALTH CONDITIONS

If you have existing health conditions such as diabetes or obesity, these can cause a significant increase in your risk of heart disease or heart attack. If you feel you want to know more about how to manage existing health conditions to lower the risk of heart disease, talk to your doctor, diabetes counsellor, nutritionist or other health care professional.

CHAPTER 9

YOU ARE YOUR NO.1 PRIORITY

"Health is a state of complete physical, mental and social well-being and not merely the absence of disease or infirmity."
World Health Organization

PRIORITISING YOU

If coming up to catch a breath is considered a luxury for you, or if it's something you don't bother to do and keep pushing through - it's time to stop and take stock!

Going into each day wondering how long you can continue at such a pace will not be a case of 'if' you will reach burnout, but when - because it will happen.

A life that involves always being in a hurry, everything being a priority, feeling that you are being pulled in all directions by your, kids, partner, boss, work colleagues or clients, is not living a healthful life.

WHAT DOES LIVING A HEALTHFUL LIFE EVEN MEAN? Here's a bit of history for you that will give you some insight. In 1948 the World Health Organisation decided that, when talking about a person's health, it should not be measured in terms of just illness or disease, but should also include physical, mental and social health.

In later years the definition was extended to include emotional, spiritual and financial health. This is because it was realised that an imbalance or upset in any one of these areas can impact a person's overall state of physical, mental and emotional wellness.

If you think about aspects of your own life, you can probably relate and understand the reasoning behind this.

You may also think as you age, that your health journey will follow the path of your parents and grandparents. It is certainly a myth that prevails, that a person will age in the same way as their immediate forebears. Many believe they are likely to develop the same diseases as a parent or grandparent did, and that their life span will be the same or similar to theirs.

This is simply not true. There are of course certain diseases and conditions that can be passed down through the genealogical line including certain cancers, cystic fibrosis, high cholesterol, haemophilia, and sickle cell anaemia, to name a few. But for most diseases, having a genetic predisposition does not mean for certain, you will get the disease.

You may inherit a familial trait for example, of weak lung function. If you smoke, you will have a higher risk of contracting a lung disease than those family members who are not smokers. Your family may have a history of high cholesterol or Type 2 diabetes but knowing this means you can do all you can to limit its impact on you by making healthy lifestyle choices.

Unless you sustain a debilitating injury or contract an unavoidable disease, you can pave your own way to a long a healthy life.

Much of the time it is the lack of knowledge or understanding that leads to poor choices or not knowing what is available to you by way of encouragement and support. The goal isn't to live for as long as you possibly can, but to have a healthy, active, purposeful and independent life, for as long as you live.

Everyone is different and will age differently. Your experience of the years leading up to menopause will be unique to you and will be significantly influenced by your lifestyle choices up to that point. It is important to be able to distinguish what are normal menopausal symptoms and natural signs of ageing, and what are not, and when you need to seek medical help.

THE THING ABOUT STRESS

Life can be stressful right? It doesn't even have to be a difficult or traumatic situation that causes you stress. It can also be caused simply by daily life events, financial worries, work pressure or not having a job. By being pulled in a million different directions. So much to do, so little time, not enough support - you know the drill.

You might not even realise you are stressed because you have normalised the speed you go through each day and the amount you fit into it. You consider your simultaneous feelings of hyper-alertness and extreme fatigue, known as 'tired but wired', to be a perfectly normal state for you, despite how debilitating it can feel.

You might already have stress-related outbursts, but put it down to just being tired or frustrated with a situation, feeling a sense of injustice or finding someone particularly annoying. It could be a normal life event that causes you stress, such as moving house, going on holiday or a celebratory event, that makes you feel anxious or overwhelmed. It is normal to feel periods of temporary stress. It's your body's way of responding and coping with a difficult or emotional situation.

However, if you feel any of the following symptoms, it is likely that it isn't an isolated emotional response weighing you down, it is deep-seated stress:

- Little things annoy, irritate or overwhelm you.
- You feel emotionally drained.
- Your body feels weary and your mind exhausted.
- You no longer want to socialise.
- You are regularly restless or anxious.
- Your mind chatter keeps you awake at night.
- You feel so tightly wound that if anyone asks you to do one more thing you are going to explode.

You might try to shrug off the initial tell-tale signs of stress, but it will soon become apparent and start to take its toll on your physical and mental health with detrimental effects.

Stress can:

- Create deep feelings of extreme emotion and vulnerability.
- Cause a strain on your heart.
- Compromise the function of your immune system.
- Cause your hair to start to fall out.
- Cause your muscles to ache.
- Result in you developing ulcers, reflux and heartburn - there is a direct link between stress and your digestive function.

Your digestive system reacts because the way you eat becomes affected when you're stressed. Either because you are in too much of a rush to eat healthily and grab whatever is quick and easy, because you use food for comfort as a coping mechanism or simply skip meals all together because you just can't be bothered to eat or your hunger cues have been dulled.

MANAGING STRESS

I have my plan all worked out to manage my stress. I aim to live on a tropical island that has beautiful weather all year round. Get regular airdrops of food, wine and books. Have no phone, internet, Facebook or other media sources and only my dog and the friendly native animals and birds for company. Sounds perfect. Nothing and no one to give me stress. I may let my husband and daughter visit sometimes but only if they agree to leave their technology devices behind. They probably won't visit.

However, back here in the real world it would likely be more beneficial to just identify the source of your stress and find ways to manage it. I know that's easier said than done, because sometimes it's hard to break it down to just one thing.

You've probably been in the scenario when something small or insignificant happened that made you completely lose your shit. This leads to you being told you are over-reacting - which makes you even more irritated - which adds another layer of stress.

Maybe you did overreact to a particular event - but because something else is gnawing away at you. It might be that the latest event was the 'straw that broke the camel's back', but as soon as the floodgates have been opened, all the pent-up emotion and frustration will come spilling out, and all those around you had better be able to swim.

Keeping things bottled up, adding layer upon layer of suppressed emotion can turn any small event into a massive conflict.

So, what can you do?

- Talk about what's troubling you when issues first arise.
- Examine the source or reason for your troubled mind.
- Get enough sleep and give yourself rest breaks.
- Be assertive without aggression. Just say No!
- Build a support network.
- Exercise regularly - this is a massive stressbuster.
- Have an outlet just for you.

And you will be welcome to come and visit me on my island for a chat and de-stress session. Bring wine.

SLEEP

It's rare to hear people complaining they've had too much sleep. Most of us are sleep-deprived at some time or other, or even all the time.

Hormones are once again to blame for sleep difficulties before and after menopause. And again, it's the declining levels of oestrogen and progesterone that are the cause of this.

Declining levels of oestrogen and progesterone, before and after menopause, bring about a chain of reactions that cause women to find it difficult to fall asleep or to stay asleep.

Older women can develop sleep apnoea, which can also interrupt sleep. It's also known that menopausal women spend less time in REM (rapid eye movement), which is the period of sleep most beneficial for you to wake up feeling rested and alert.

There are other hormones at play too. Too high serotonin levels can be a factor of restless sleep, as can an over-active thyroid. The hormonal upheaval going on in middle age means that the imbalance of one hormone has a knock-on effect on other hormones - which retaliate by trying to redress the balance - but instead… chaos ensues!

The same activities to promote sleep still apply as you get older, just as they did in your younger years, such as:

- Keeping a regular sleep schedule.
- Relaxing in the hours leading up to bedtime.
- Avoiding caffeine and alcohol from late afternoon.
- Avoiding screens in the bedroom that give off light - phone, television.
- Keeping a regular exercise routine.

- Engaging in stimulating activities during the day to keep you awake.
- Taking a short nap, if the need arises - but no more than an hour.
- Eating light meals.
- Not eating close to bedtime.
- Managing stress.
- Trying homeopathy or, with professional advice - hormonal treatments.

You may feel tired beyond what is usual for you, feel your energy is low, or be experiencing dizzy spells, headaches and weak muscles. The consequences of poor sleep due to the effects of the pervading hormonal meltdown can result in chronic fatigue. You may also be experiencing mood swings and feelings of aggression and irritability.

These feelings are all normal side effects of the age-related decrease in progesterone, but if fatigue persists or becomes too intense, you may benefit from a consultation with your doctor.

You may also have heard or believe that you need less sleep as you age. This is yet another myth. There is no evidence to support this. Adults require, on average, between seven and nine hours of sleep each night, although the exact number of hours will vary from person to person. Some might need only six hours, others can't function unless they have ten, but age has no bearing on this.

It's likely this myth is passed around because aging and retired people may have a nap during the day, which means they will sleep less overnight. It's not that aging people need less sleep, but some find that they just can't stay asleep because of aching joints, or they just need to get up to pee more often!

Regardless, these interruptions can cause disturbed sleep patterns that may amount to less sleep, but it isn't because older people need less of it.

ALONE – TO BE OR NOT TO BE

For some women, having time alone means going to the hairdresser, getting your nails done or maybe a massage. Alone time might also mean time away from the routines and responsibilities of everyday life by catching up with friends for coffee or a glass of wine or going on a shopping trip. All excellent pursuits that are wholeheartedly encouraged. But what about time totally to, and by yourself?

Sometimes you just need time to think and be completely on your own; a total break from dealing with the tedium of everyday routines. It's quite normal to want to get away, switch off your phone, ignore messages and not be pestered with what sometimes feels like trivial dialogue, petty family squabbles or workplace bitching.

Having time on your own is essential, so don't feel guilty about wanting it.

I know from personal experience, that you can sometimes feel that the noise in your head is going to make it explode. You can feel crazy and wish someone would just flick the switch and make everything be still and silent, just while you gather your thoughts and try to draw on some inner calm.

It can be difficult to achieve this in an ever-evolving world of technology, social media interactions and the constant bombardment of information. Persistent pings, dings, tunes, bells and bloody whistles from phones and computers.

You might think scrolling your social media is having alone time. Granted it can be fun and engaging, but there is so much absolute twaddle put up by people that it's easy to get irritated and feel compelled to let some half-wit know they are behaving like a moron.

And before you know it you find yourself getting into a keyboard stoush. If this is you, give yourself a time out. There might be no-one physically there, but you are still giving others far too much mental and emotional headspace.

Having time for and by yourself means alone. No outside influence, noise or distractions, just you, giving your body, mind, heart and soul, time and opportunity to recharge and reset. You can't do that in the hustle and bustle of everyday life.

I really enjoy time on my own. I'm extremely comfortable being by myself. In fact, me and myself have sorted out quite a lot of shit together when there is no outside influence. Peace and quiet is bliss. I always say that if I want noise, I'll make it myself - and I do when the mood takes me which, if I'm honest, is often.

There are, however, many women, who simply find the prospect of being alone daunting. They don't feel comfortable in their own company. They find the quietness is deafening and the solitude overwhelming.

There are many reasons someone might not want to be alone:

- They fear being alone.
- It can make them feel sad, anxious or lonely.
- They can't appreciate that being alone has benefits.
- They don't know what to do with themselves when alone.
- They feel bored and restless.
- They find it too overwhelming to be alone with their thoughts and can only think about past trauma, current troubles or unresolved issues.
- Some need to be around other people to feel secure or validated.
- Others may have existing mental health conditions that are exacerbated by being alone.

Perhaps you can relate to some of these. If so, take it one step at a time. Think of activities you can do on your own. Practise just sitting on your own and quieting your mind chatter for short periods. Switch off the television, log out of Facebook and online games. Lose yourself in a good book, puzzle, cross-stitch, whatever it is you like to do. Just enjoy the quiet.

Your strength comes from inside you, nurture that and know you are strong and self-sufficient, and that being on your own is a safe place. Sometimes life can beat you up or slap you down, sap your confidence and your belief in yourself. Knowing how you can find calm, comfort and peace in the safety of your own company, in your own sense of self, will allow you to reassess, revive and recover, and continue to live in a meaningful way.

The other side of the coin is that many women prefer to spend most of their time on their own. They choose to be and are happy to. They don't feel the need to always have company and neither invite it in, nor seek it out. They can generate their own entertainment, activities, and hobbies.

They like their own company. They enjoy extended time alone to free their mind, consider their aspirations and set goals or just relax without having any outside interference or influence. Being comfortable in your own skin, enjoying your own time and company is a perfectly healthy state of mind if it brings you peace and keeps you positive.

But another flip of the coin can reveal a less shiny side to this. If you are choosing to be alone because you live with perpetual apathy, you just drift aimlessly day to day, achieving nothing, not wanting to go anywhere or do anything - you need to accept that this is not a healthy state of mind.

People with these behaviours are usually highly stressed, frequently reactive, focus on negativity and are unable to cope with day-to-day situations. This shutting down and shutting out is a clear sign of withdrawal and depression. Sadly, such people have normalised their behaviour and see it as perfectly healthy state of mind for them to be in.

They will disagree, argue and insist it is not a problem. They won't seek help or even consider that they need it. If you know someone like this, don't try and force them into anything they don't want to do. You don't want to make them feel like they want to become even further isolated because of what they will perceive as your interference.

For those of you who have crazy busy lives, whose 'to-do' list is always a mile long, who always needs to be somewhere, meet someone, cook, clean, shop... you get my drift. I say to you just stop and breathe.

Reassess your priorities and factor in some time for yourself every single day. Set the intent. Mark it in your calendar as a personal appointment, and don't be distracted or guilted into giving that time to someone or something else.

Challenge yourself to take 20-30 minutes each day to be completely on your own. Do what you need to do to get precious time alone. Get out into nature and absorb the peace around you. Go for a drive on a country road, find a spot by water and sit under a tree and just ponder the things that are most important to you.

Even if you don't want to go anywhere, just remove yourself from noise, people, technology, get a coffee or glass of wine, pick up a book or just sit quietly. For absolutely everyone, meaningful alone time is an essential coping mechanism giving you space to refocus and reenergise. Your mental health will thank you.

Good overall health always comes back down to the basics. And yes, I know you've heard this many times before but I'm going to say it again anyway and it won't be for the last time before the end of this book:

- Get enough sleep.
- Eat regularly and make sure you eat good food and stay hydrated.
- Exercise your body and your mind.
- Take time out to be alone and sit in quiet reflection.
- Take part in mindful meditation to give your brain the chance to clear.
- Give your body the means to relax, rejuvenate and replenish.

HOW HEALTHY ARE YOUR RELATIONSHIPS?

So, from being completely alone to mixing with other people. Even the most insular of introverts, unless a total recluse, cannot generally help having relationships with others as they move through aspects of their daily life.

We all know people. Mix with people - live, work, socialise, interact at various levels and give our time, energy and emotion to others. Do you ever assess those relationships and consider how much of yourself you invest in them or what they mean to you?

You clearly know the importance of maintaining a healthy relationship with your partner, children, extended family, friends and co-workers. It's what makes our existence meaningful and it's vital to our own sense of health and wellbeing.

Unhealthy relationships can take a huge toll on your mental and physical health. It can lead to stress, depression, high blood pressure and decreased immune system, to name just a few. On a base level they can leave you hurt, angry, frustrated, disappointed, mega pissed off and sometimes murderous! These people are draining your life blood and your peace of mind. And not worth going to jail for!

If any relationship you have, whether a close family member or a casual Facebook friend, is causing negativity in any part of your life, it's time to take a good, hard look at that relationship and the reason you are allowing them to occupy such a big place in your heart and mind.

There may be someone in your life who causes you to think negative thoughts about yourself and have you doubt your worth. Do not let this person inside your head. Nothing and no one should diminish your feelings or crush your confidence. Anyone who causes you to feel in any way inferior or inadequate does not have your happiness at heart and does not deserve a place in it.

Close personal relationships should be supportive and kind and bring you joy, give you confidence, feelings of trust and security. If any of them bring anything less than this, it's time to review why you keep them in your life. Assess the relationships you have. Make peace where you need to and cut ties with those who are negative soul sucking leeches, those that make you miserable and those who challenge your feelings of mental or emotional balance.

Cull your Facebook 'friends' list and surround yourself only with people who have proved themselves to be worthy of being in your life. As you age, the quality of your friends becomes much more important than the quantity.

Strong, mutually respectful relationships are linked to your physical, mental, emotional, spiritual and social wellbeing. Surround yourself with only those who love, support and respect you. Never allow yourself to be a push-over. As you move through your advancing years, flex some muscle and be a force to be reckoned with.

Chapter 10

One Step Beyond!

Life After Menopause

Here we are - menopause. I mean actual menopause. Up to now we have mainly spoken about menopause in terms of the transitional phase, or 'perimenopause', the symptoms and the upheaval, but now here you are at the main event.

The official marker that you have reached menopause is when you have gone a continuous 12-months without having a period.

For all the misery that occurs in the years up to this point, all the hormonal changes and all the discomfort that comes with it, reaching menopause seems like a bit of a non-event. Of course, it means no more periods, which is a relief. Once a woman's desire to become pregnant has passed, she is no doubt more than happy to see the end of this monthly annoyance. Even so, it seems like an inadequate final bow for all the years of biological upheaval women experience to get to this point.

You can't mark the day to throw a party to celebrate or commiserate - depending on how your feel about it - because unless you've been keeping track of the dates and ticking off the months, your entry into menopause will likely be overlooked. However, for biological, societal and medical purposes you have now graduated to a new column marked 'post-menopause', and this is where you will stay, through to the end of your life.

You may suddenly become aware that, having reached this milestone, you are more than half-way through your life. You shouldn't let this engender feelings of gloom and doom or the beginning of the end! Once upon a time, 55 was the average years of a woman's life, therefore reaching menopause signified being near to death. The extended lifespan for today's woman is much higher and now menopause is just a tick in the box before you move on to the next 30+ years.

Embrace life after menopause. The Grim Reaper is not going to come knocking any time soon.

Look on this time as another new beginning, that you should embrace with plans, goals, hope and enthusiasm. Keep a positive and open mind. I know I have drawn your attention to many of the downsides of getting older, but instead of feeling threatened by it, use the knowledge to enhance your awareness and improve your lifestyle. Take the opportunity to reassess your habits and daily life to create a more healthful one.

Women can live healthily well into their eighties and even nineties, meaning you can enjoy nearly as many years of life after menopause as you had before it. It's for this reason you need to keep looking after yourself, set new health goals and do everything you can to ensure you are living well.

That said, you're not quite out of the woods regarding the effects of hormone and vitamin depletion. In the post-menopause stage, you may still have to contend with some of the symptoms that you did during perimenopause. Hot flushes, for example, are still very common and the hormone deficiencies you will now be experiencing may start to have more noticeable consequences. We spoke earlier about these deficiencies that can affect your bones, muscles, heart and other internal organs, as well as your general ability to function as well as you once did. You may start to experience other health issues too.

But you are not going to wake up on the morning of your 60th birthday and suddenly find you have lost all your faculties. That happens the day after your party - but can most likely be attributed to too much of the falling down juice.

As ageing progresses, a number of unavoidable characteristics are associated with it. Hearing loss, impaired vision, forgetfulness and others. You can't stop the ageing process, but you can influence the rate at which the symptoms of ageing present themselves.

You will no doubt have heard many tales of what to expect as you age. Some of it will be fact, some will be age-old myths based on generational stereotyping and others are simply not true. Myths regarding life after menopause are believed by many women and creates unfounded fears for what life ahead holds for them. Let's have a look at some of the most common myths and debunk them once and for all!

I'm Worried About Becoming Forgetful

Forgetfulness is not uncommon and happens at all ages throughout our lives, especially when our minds are over-worked and over-tired. We've been through the forgetful teenager and baby brain stages, the stressful job, juggling work/life/family/social/finances. Forgetting things is not surprising when you have mental overload.

Becoming forgetful and easily confused is a fear that many people have of ageing. As time passes you may find that the extent of your memory loss starts to disrupt your day-to-day living. You may experience symptoms such as feeling confused with time or a place or feeling you are missing parts of conversations because you can't process the words fast enough.

You can do much to help yourself to remember things - write things down, leave yourself a note, keep a paper diary or use an online calendar. Devise a way that works for you to help you to remember. There is also plenty you can do to improve your memory. Experts in these matters recommend doing mental agility exercises and activities that challenge your brain and keep you mentally alert.

In some people, forgetfulness can be a sign of senility, Alzheimer's or other type of dementia, and is most common from the age of 65. Senility and dementia are not the same, and nor are dementia and Alzheimer's, despite all these terms often being used interchangeably.

Symptoms of senility can be mild and affect your memory and concentration. It is not a disease; it is just a natural part of ageing and is no longer considered a medical condition.

Alzheimer's is a distinct and progressive condition that causes severe mental regression and impaired daily function. There are a number of categories of Alzheimer's but, despite some genetic components running in families, only early-onset Alzheimer's is considered an inherited disease.

Dementia is the over-arching term used in the medical profession to describe and encompass various cognitive disease characteristics that cause mental decline.

It's important to know that cognitive decline does not happen to everyone just because they are getting older. Nor does it mean that because there is a history of dementia in your family, that you too will be affected. Factors such as your environment, medical conditions and other lifestyle factors play a significant part in determining the likelihood.

You can in fact live well into your nineties with very little mental decline, so don't go worrying about something that may never happen to you. If you do experience symptoms you no longer feel are 'normal' for you, or a loved one mentions that you regularly appear confused, you may wish to seek professional advice.

It's Too Difficult To Learn New Things When You Get Older

Because the myth prevails that all older adults somehow become mentally impaired when they reach a certain age, it's assumed that learning new things is not an option for them. This is of course rubbish.

You can teach an old dog new tricks. Older people, including very old people are more than capable of learning new tricks too. In fact, learning new things and keeping yourself mentally active is a totally positive step in slowing down mental decline. Older people have many intellectual, practical, social and logical reasoning skills from years of living life. They have a lot they can teach, a lot they can still learn and the capacity to do both, if they wish.

The 2024 Senior Australian of the Year recipient was Bronwyn Herbert. At the age of 40 she first graduated from university with a bachelor's degree in social work. At 61 she earned her Master's. She retired as a social worker at the age of 81 and went on to complete her PhD at the age of 90.

Dr Herbert's work, especially around homelessness and its effect on children, is said to have "changed countless lives nationally and contributed to a better understanding of homelessness and how to break the cycle".

Okay, my absolute respect for this woman aside, let's take a minute. Not for one second am I suggesting you rush out and enrol in a university degree. My point here is that you should never, ever believe you are too old to learn or take up something new, a hobby, get creative or start whatever it is you have always wanted to do. I qualified as a dog groomer when I was aged 64 and groomed local dogs for a few years. Why? Because I wanted to.

What you do doesn't have to be a job or something mind-blowing, just mind-stretching, like reading, doing crosswords or other puzzles, writing a book, your memoirs, learning another language or picking up an instrument. Not because you want to become a literary or academic genius or intend to go on your country's Got Talent show, but because you want to remain as mentally agile for as long as possible. Your brain loves and thrives on knowledge. Keep feeding it!

OLDER PEOPLE DON'T HAVE SEX

Don't they? Oh, okay. How many of us didn't get that memo? It's certainly a thing that younger people think, that once you get to a certain age you no longer engage in sexual or intimate activities. In their words, they are 'grossed out' at the thought of it - especially if you're over 50.

Sex is a very personal thing. It generates physical and emotional feelings, which are not of course, specifically age-related. Some older women may have very active sex lives, whilst others may no longer have sex at all. There are many reasons an older, or any woman for that matter, may no longer be interested in or participate in sexual activities.

Through the transitional phase and following menopause, the symptoms of a woman's warring hormones are likely to make her feel like sex is not on her list of priorities. Or, as hormones fluctuate, she may well become very interested in sex.

As you age, sex for a woman may become painful. That's because the natural lubrication of your vagina becomes dryer and the walls thinner. It can be either slow to lubricate or it just doesn't. When sex is painful it doesn't make for enthusiastic participation. Talk to your partner and work out how you can still be there for each other sexually and still make it pleasurable for you both.

There are of course other reasons why sex is difficult, uncomfortable or even a chore. If you are living with pain, arthritis, joint problems, depression - all these conditions can lead to sleepless nights, fatigue or exhaustion, leaving you little enthusiasm or energy for horizontal gymnastics.

If you and your partner are still having a healthy sexual relationship, that's great. If one or both of you are no longer comfortable about it, an open and honest conversation between you will help.

You may not be aware, but men also go through a process called 'andropause'. This is similar to menopause and occurs when male levels of testosterone start to deplete as they age. They don't have symptoms of menopause like women do, but sex may become more difficult in later life for them too.

Depending on how important this aspect of your relationship is to you both as you age, there are number of over-the-counter lubricants or other treatments you can both try, or you can seek external advice from a sexual health professional.

You can have love and intimacy without sex. You can't have understanding and respect for each other's feelings or discomfort without meaningful discussion. The most important thing is to talk about it.

Just an aside note about andropause. Most men don't know this happens to them. Don't tell them. If they know that it happens there is no doubt they will imagine symptoms far worse than anything you experience in menopause - it will be the hormone equivalent of man flu! Don't say you weren't warned.

I'm Worried About Becoming Weak And Frail

This is a concern for many. Nobody wants to have a drastically reduced quality of life or find they can no longer function independently. Whether this happens or not can be largely up to you.

Like mental decline, weakness and frailty is not an inevitable condition of ageing.

How you live your life up to perimenopause, during transition and beyond menopause, is the key to combating many of the ills that ageing brings. We have talked about accepting there are some things you don't have control over, but that's not what we are focussing on here. The focus is on what you *can* do for yourself to achieve better health and longevity, not what you can't.

Being active, eating a healthy balanced diet, and staying socially connected are all ways that you can improve your health and defer dependency, no matter what age you are.

CHAPTER 11

REFLECT, REASSESS, RECREATE

"If you don't like where you are, move.
You're not a tree."
Jim Rohn, Motivational Speaker

CHANGE CAN BE BETTER THAN A REST!
It is common for women to get to middle age and find
themselves reflecting on the years gone by and feel this is
'crunch' time. Reaching the cross-roads of your life means
you are standing at a point from where you can choose
the direction you now want your life to go - or stay where
you are. If you are not currently living the life you want,
it's no use acknowledging that to yourself and then doing
nothing about it.

Ask yourself the questions: Am I happy, satisfied and content or am I miserable, frustrated and disillusioned? Am I thriving or in a rut? Happy at work or simply tolerating the daily grind to pay the bills?

You have the choice to continue as you are or make a change. You've reached the middle of your life and what happens next is entirely up to you. Don't see this as being the end of something. It isn't, it's the start of some new and amazing opportunities - so take them, seek them out or create them for yourself.

If you want to make a change and are ready to do that, what or who is holding you back from living the life you want, the life you worked for and feel you earned, the one you deserve? Is it something in your current life, in your past, or does the future concern you so much you don't plan for it, you just live one day at a time?

We all have commitments and yes, obligations too, that we can't just walk away from, but that doesn't mean you can't plan and work towards new pathways to change your job, move to a different town, go travelling - whatever it is that will give you purpose and goals to set your sights on.

Every woman is different and each of us starts the next decade of life in the frame of mind crafted by her previous years on this earth. I personally feel that between the ages of 40 and 50 women start to reassess their life in a more philosophical way. It's probably universal that at the start of every new decade, a woman wonders what she wants to achieve in the future and at the same time, wonders where the hell the last decade went.

Turning 50 is a little bit different. Up to this point you are ticking off life's milestones and suddenly, here you are - at menopause. The next age milestone after this is 60. At 40, turning 60 seemed a long way away, at 50 it's looming over the horizon, it's the next stop!

Society deems you to be old at 60. Horror of all horrors, you get your Seniors Card! Mine came through the post a week after my 60th birthday. I remember opening it and laughingly throwing it in a drawer thinking - 'bloody cheek - how rude!' I wasn't ready to be considered 'senior'; my mind hadn't caught up with that yet. I've mellowed since then. You get discounts on stuff with a Seniors Card! So, I thought what the hell, don't be pissy, embrace the positives.

Whether you like it or not, here you are and it's time to choose. You can flop into apathy, do nothing and let the rest of your life roll by without plan or purpose. Or you can throw yourself into it with energy and enthusiasm and create some of your best memories yet.

You can decide that there's no point in starting any exercise or healthy lifestyle changes at your age and wait until you fall into the pit of avoidable dependency. Or you can be fit - physically, mentally and emotionally, and go into the second half of your life, independently and on your own terms in great health.

You choose.

I hope that you welcome this juncture and embrace this time of your life to embark on a journey of purpose, self-discovery and growth. Your 50s and 60s can be your best years of your life. Whilst you still have years in front of you, the best years can always be ahead. It's a new era of promise and opportunity.

You may have been a late starter on the children front like me, but by the time you are 60 they will be independent enough for you to not worry so much about being physically there for them all the time. For most women over 60, their children will have long flown the nest.

You can develop a new sense of freedom, do the things you always said you couldn't do because of your responsibilities, kids and work. How many times did you say, you would do that, or go there, take up this hobby, learn something new or even go travelling with a partner or friend, or by yourself. You can do all that now. The possibilities are endless. No more excuses. Make changes *to* your life and see a difference *in* your life.

But what is it you need to do to take the plunge, to make that decision and just do it? Why do some of us hesitate?

WILLPOWER V MOTIVATION

"It's not that some people have the willpower and some don't. It's that some people are ready to change, and others are not."
James Gordon

All the reasons we gave ourselves for why we couldn't follow our dreams or achieve our own personal goals have faded into the background. You are now free to take the next step. And yet here you are, on the precipice of new independence, adventure and growth - but too fearful to take the leap.

Why is that? For an explanation I am going to draw on dialogue that I usually use when talking to my weight loss clients. Nearly every woman I have ever coached told me that they had not been successful in previous attempts to lose weight because they didn't have the willpower. By that they meant they couldn't stay committed.

But that's not what willpower is. If you set out on a path to do something, and you don't achieve it, it's not willpower you lack, it's motivation.

Willpower relates to the control you apply to yourself to actually do it, and it is something you have absolute control over. Everyone has the willpower, but not everyone is motivated to use it.

Motivation is a combination of the reasons you want to do something, your purpose whilst doing it, what your end goal is – what you want to achieve and why it's important to you.

Staying committed to continue towards your goal is not about willpower. It's about motivation. Why do you want to lose weight, why do you want to change your job, why do you want to travel? Motivation is driven by having a compelling reason for wanting to achieve something.

To confirm whether you are sufficiently motivated to do something, the reason you are doing it should make you feel emotional, it should stir something inside you whenever you think about it. If you don't feel those stirrings, your reasons for wishing to achieve it aren't going to be strong enough. Without the emotion, you won't be motivated to carry it through. You need to find and believe in that reason. Keep digging, it's in there. If it's not, ask yourself the question 'is what I'm striving for, really what I want', then answer yourself honestly.

SELF-PERPETUATING CYCLE OR SELF-FULFILLING PROPHECY

A self-perpetuating cycle is when an event, or chain of events, keep repeating itself. It seems impossible to break the chain because the issue appears to have taken on a life of its own, and it just keeps going round, and round again.

What I mean by this is, if you have had a situation in your life that turned out to be a negative experience, every time you approach a similar situation, your subconscious will throw up all the negativity from that previous experience. These feelings and the negative energy you put out will 'self-perpetuate' a negative outcome, over and over again.

I gave the example earlier of my maths teacher who told me I was stupid. He told me I would fail. And I did. I did extremely poorly in all my school exams. I was even late for one exam, English Literature, which was by far my best subject. I had been really worried about failing this exam as it was the only subject I believed I was good at; because I arrived so late, I wasn't allowed into the exam and therefore marked as a fail. I don't recall that I was deliberately late but I have wondered if I sub-consciously self-sabotaged. After all, if I didn't take the exam I couldn't fail it. To have taken the exam and failed would have confirmed to me that I really was stupid and Mr. Nasty Arse the maths teacher would have been right all along.

I wasn't surprised or disappointed I did so badly in all my exams, because it was exactly what I expected; it's what I believed others expected, that I just wasn't good enough to have done any better.

You can be discouraged from doing something and believe something that isn't necessarily true because of a past experience, without you even realising that it had such a profound effect on you.

Stop the cycle, break the chain - apply any other idiom you like, but become aware of the patterns in your behaviour that drive your negative thoughts in a given situation. Accept that you are pressing your own self-destruct button with your negative self-talk and lack of belief in yourself. Challenge the root cause of your feelings. Why do you think like you do? Who or what brought about this negativity?

Think of what you can put in place to overcome this, what coping mechanisms you can use. If necessary, speak to a counsellor who may be able to help you to work through the issue that spawned the negativity. Continuing to allow the negativity to have an ongoing hold on you will have a detrimental effect on your long-term mental and emotional health.

A self-fulfilling prophecy sounds like it is the same as above but, although similar, and interchanged in some descriptions, there are differences. The main one is that it is not attached to a recurring situation that always ends with the same negative result because you went into it believing it would.

Self-fulfilling prophecy has a more positive aura. It's about putting positivity out into the universe, if you are of the mind to use this expression. Believing good things will happen will exert your willpower, uplift your motivation levels and bring about an overall positive attachment to the situation.

A self-fulfilling prophecy occurs when our own underlying or subconscious expectations influence the actions we take which, when built on, brings the achievements you had set your sights on. My university professor challenged me to challenge myself. He inspired me to believe in myself to the point that I didn't for one second believe I could fail. I was 100% committed to see the course through to the end, no matter how tough it got, to achieve my goal. I kept telling myself all the things I would achieve in the short and long term and kept pushing through, and I succeeded.

I've said it a few times that you don't need to go to university to be successful, but for me, making that decision created an unforeseen opportunity and benefits. Had I not gone to university, we would not have met the criteria to emigrate to New Zealand from the UK in 2001.

I had no idea when I decided to go to university that I would emigrate. It was a decision made after Ivan and I had married and had our daughter. To qualify for a visa you need a specific number of 'points' to satisfy the NZ immigration criteria. Without the points for having a degree, we would never have secured enough points to have moved there, and from there to Australia five years later. So that was just a happy aside.

Believing you can, will inspire you towards positive thoughts, outlook and actions that will bring about your own self-fulfilment.

STEP INTO YOUR DISCOMFORT ZONE

You might think this title is arse about face, but it isn't. It is exactly what I am asking you to do. I have often wondered what the phrase as it is usually said, 'step out of your comfort zone', is meant to achieve. I think it's supposed to motivate you to take on a challenge head-on, but the phrase itself sets you up for failure. It presents a feeling of dread that you are stepping into a situation you will find difficult, intimidating, nerve-racking, fearful or unpleasant. It conjures feelings of not being in control, powerless, that whatever happens out of your figurative 'comfort zone' will be something that is unfamiliar to you, something you won't like and there is nothing you can do about it.

We've talked about changing the narrative before and this is another occasion to do that. By stepping _**into**_ your _**dis**_comfort zone, you are immediately telling yourself that you are ready to deal with it. Most people won't deliberately choose to be uncomfortable, so turn the negative into a positive.

Next time you are faced with a situation that is alien to you, or you know makes you uncomfortable, change the narrative to inspire you, see it as an opportunity for growth. Acknowledge that the situation you are about to go into may not be the most pleasant or the most comfortable of situations - but approach it with confidence and not trepidation.

You might not be able to control the situation, but you can prepare yourself to decisively respond to it. You can control how you approach it, step into it, deal with it and how you come out of the other side. Brace yourself for what might be a rough time and prepare yourself accordingly. There is always the chance that, as often happens, things turn out not nearly as bad as you envisioned.

REGRET NOTHING!

This is easier said than done sometimes. It's unfortunate that regret is one of those emotions that can eat you up from the inside out for months and even years. The decisions that you made in the past not only affected you at the time you made them but can continue to affect you now. They can make you feel miserable or uneasy. You might avoid going somewhere you used to go, or meeting someone you used to know, for fear of past mistakes being resurrected that you would rather not be reminded of.

We've explored a lot about the impact middle age can have on a woman, not least that it precipitates a journey of reflection that can resurface past events, and not all of them memorable in a good way.

Spending too much time in your past and dwelling on unfulfilled dreams, periods of sadness or the shame of a lingering regret for things you either did, or didn't do, are obstacles to present and future happiness, and peace of mind.

If you are harbouring regret for past actions or inactions, you are creating a whole host of negativity that can affect your mental state and your overall sense of wellbeing.

I'd not be being honest if I said I didn't have pangs of remorse for poor decisions I made in the past. Most of the time I don't think about them at all, and then one little thing, a word, a name, or a song, will drag a memory back to the fore and it might torment me for a while. I have worked hard on myself to reconcile that who I was and how I behaved in previous incarnations, is not who I am now. I repeatedly made poor choices - usually when alcohol was involved, which fed my cycle of low self-esteem. After I moved away from that environment I began to figure out who I really wanted to be and what I wanted to achieve.

It was at this time, in my mid-thirties, that I knew I had to change my life or live the same one unhappily for the rest of it. I'm not going to pretend that it was easy to change. After leaving the Army I made some of the hardest decisions of my life, mentally, physically and emotionally. But without a doubt, it was worth it.

I have no regrets and feel grateful that I found the strength to shake off the old mantel and put on another one, not one that was completely undamaged, but certainly less bruised.

By the time you reach middle age, you have two periods of life left to live. The here and now, and the future - both of which are yours to create. You can't change what has gone before but you can learn from it. There is no benefit to wishing you had done something differently, at the time you didn't, so put it away somewhere, in a metaphorical sealed box in your mind. Write 'the past' on it and leave it there, to gather cobwebs.

I have, for as long as I can remember, compartmentalised and 'boxed up' parts of my past life. I have read a bit around this subject - it is said to be an unhealthy, dissociative trait, that it is often used as a coping or defence mechanism.

This was based on the assertion that people box up situations that they are afraid to deal with and to protect themselves emotionally. It also said that those who do this set themselves on a self-perpetuating cycle and would continue to repeat past mistakes.

I have given a lot of thought to this, and since honesty is always the best policy, I concede that there is some truth to this from my own perspective. However, whilst I agree in part, it failed to address the liberating feeling of leaving something behind. I have 'boxed' people, situations, whole eras. Not necessarily because they made me sad or that I harbour bad or negative feelings about them, or that I no longer care about them - but because they no longer hold a part of me that needs them to be in my life as it is now. Then was then, this is now.

Sometimes a good memory stirs and I figuratively unpack a box of nostalgic moments. I allow myself to wallow there, remembering the laughs, the fun, the great people, the scrapes we got into, and those we talked ourselves out of.

And I love it. I savour it for a while and then I box it back up and check it back into the library in my mind, ready to take out another day if I choose.

Nostalgia can be wonderfully positive or crushingly negative. By definition, it occurred in the past. And, if the experience was a bad one, that is where you should leave it. The past can't be changed and it doesn't need to be still living in your heart and mind in the present or in the future.

If you have been giving a front row seat in your head to negative occurrences from your past, challenge yourself to detach from the emotion that fuels your regret. Focus on all the good things you have done since that time and put your energy into creating the future you want rather than a past you can't change. Once you do this, peace of mind and a state of calm will prevail. If you really feel like you can't achieve this, don't be afraid to seek professional help.

CHAPTER 12

THE IMPORTANCE OF YOU - REVISITED

"I'm not sure If I'm walking through life anymore, or if life is just walking through me."
R.K Nightingale, Writer, Poet

The aim throughout this book has been to share with you what I believe to be the fundamental principles of good health; physical, mental and emotional, as you age.

Some of the key messages in the book are worth revisiting, particularly around:

- Self-care and psychological self-preservation.
- Nutrition and exercise.

SELF-CARE AND PSYCHOLOGICAL SELF-PRESERVATION

Grab a coffee and find somewhere quiet where you will be uninterrupted and think about what resonated with you the most, as you went through this book.

How good do you consider your overall health? This includes physical, mental, social, emotional, spiritual and financial matters. How healthy are your relationships and how happy are you with the way people treat you, and the way you treat others? It's a two-way street.

Use the blank pages at the end of this chapter to write down some key points, ready to construct and prioritise an action plan.

Which areas of your life could do with an overhaul and how will you decide what needs to be done?

Reflect on your current lifestyle. You don't necessarily need to be 'living the dream' but you do need to have purpose and be striving to be happy.

Reassess all aspects of your life. Identify what is no longer contributing to your wellbeing or is stopping you from realising your potential.

Recreate your narrative. You can't change the past but can create your future. If you are not happy in a situation, change it. I have said it previously - you will never be too old, and it will never be too late.

Don't try to do everything at once. Adopt an incremental change strategy, make one small change, then another and another. Build on the previous achievement - not only will it be easier to manage, it will also serve to encourage and motivate you to continue.

Nutrition and Exercise

I have covered a lot of detail on these subjects throughout the book and in specific detail in Chapters 7 and 8. When I read it back, I wish I could find a way to say it in a more compelling, more persuasive, more convincing way, that maintaining good nutrition and staying active are the most vital factors of good health as you age - factors that are totally within your control.

I get frustrated that so many women don't believe this or don't want to believe it. They want to become healthy, lose weight and have more energy. But they want it to happen quickly and easily, and to make as little personal effort as possible to achieve it. That's not how it works. When did anything worth having come about without effort or sacrifice?

There is some repetition coming up, but I make no apologies for it. No harm will come from hearing a message multiple times to engrain it.

In fact, my message hasn't changed since I first started my nutrition coaching many years ago. Any weight loss idea that is marketed as no effort, no hunger, no exercise required, fat drops off, inject yourself with this drug or take a pill, is likely to be no bloody good for you and certainly won't benefit you in the long term. You will no doubt lose weight using these methods, because believe it or not, losing weight isn't the most difficult part.

The most difficult part is committing yourself to learning how to balance your food intake nutritionally and proportionally, and when you have achieved this, you will be able to keep the weight off for the rest of your life. To do this requires a total overhaul of your habits and an absolute shift in your mindset. There was no magic wand when we were working our way through all the diet fads of the 70s and 80s and beyond, and there isn't now.

I'm still perplexed that, no matter how many decades go by, how much money a woman spent during her weight-on-weight-off yo-yo years, how many times she fails and fails again, the message does not sink in - that there is no such thing as a sustainable quick fix.

I'll never give up trying to get the message through though. I'll keep beating my drum that a balanced diet of the right food in the right quantities from across the food groups, and some daily exercise activity, is the only healthy, long-term way to lose weight, keep weight off and stay healthy into old age.

We are not talking extremes. I am not super-strict with myself. I apply a 'don't deprive' and 'everything in moderation' approach. You do have to accept a few irritating anomalies around food groups though. For example, grapes are fruit, they are healthy, and you can eat them regularly. Wine on the other hand is made from grapes, but it is not a fruit. Can you drink as much wine as you want and remain healthy? No. There is no honour in the food kingdom. Believe me, there's no-one more appalled at this injustice than me.

To re-emphasise the relevance of good nutrition and the importance of maintaining a healthy weight as you age, I am going to expand a little more on what was given in previous chapters. I want this information to be the last message in the book so that it remains fresh in your mind.

By incorporating the healthy food options below into your diet you will be off to a great start to feed your brain, heart, muscles and bones the nutrition they need, via a healthy well-functioning digestive system.

Let's start with that big lump of grey and white matter inside your head.

BRAIN FOOD

You will have heard of antioxidants, and that foods rich in antioxidants are the key to mental clarity. If you incorporate these foods into your diet, you will rival Einstein before you know it. Maybe not, but you will benefit greatly.

- Strawberries, raspberries, blueberries, cherries.
- Dark leafy greens, carrots, pumpkin, avocados, beetroot.
- Pecans, walnuts.
- Kidney beans, black beans.
- Oily fish - rich in Omega-3 - Salmon, mackerel, sardines.
- Herbs and spices - turmeric, basil, oregano, ginger,cinnamon.

Eat Your Heart Healthy

You don't need me to tell you how important your heart is. It's not enough to feel comforted that you can still feel it beating, that just means you're not dead! For your heart to work optimally, to keep pumping blood around your body, deliver hormones and nutrients to your cells, keep your lungs oxygenated, remove waste to the organs that are going to deal with it and maintain a healthy blood pressure - it needs your help. And the way you do it is to feed it what it needs for it to play nice.

Include the following in your diet:

- Vegetables - leafy greens, spinach, cabbage, broccoli, carrots.
- Fruit - bananas, apples, oranges, pears, prunes, grapes.
- Whole grains such as brown rice and wholegrain bread.
- Dairy including milk, cheese and yogurt but avoid saturated fat.
- Protein - include oily fish - salmon and tuna, lean cuts of meat and poultry, eggs, nuts and seeds, legumes and tofu.
- Healthy fats, olive oil sunflower oil, walnuts, almonds and avocados.

Reduce the amount of sodium/salt in and on your food. Be especially careful of packaged and processed foods and frozen ready meals, as many are high in sodium added sugars and other preservatives.

If you have high cholesterol or there is a history of high cholesterol in your family, you will need to be particularly mindful, especially with the fats and sugars that you eat. Regular checks of your cholesterol levels through a simple blood test will keep you on track to maintaining healthy levels. You doctor can refer you.

STRENGTHENING BONES

You will have had it drummed into you as a child that you needed to drink your milk to give you strong bones. Obviously over-simplified for children but not incorrect.

You can slow down the impact of bone degeneration by eating well and ensuring you get enough calcium and Vitamin D in your diet. Like most recipes for success, small changes over time will instil good habits that your bones will love you for. You won't see the difference, but you will most definitely feel it.

Check how many of these calcium rich 'bone foods' you currently include in your diet:

- Green, leafy vegetables - broccoli, cabbage.
- Fruit (fresh).
- Nuts (not salted).
- Legumes (peas, kidney beans, black beans, chickpeas, lentils).
- Soya beans.
- Fish (including tinned salmon and tuna - plain or herb, not the ones with the yucky and questionable sauces and flavourings).
- Dairy (milk, cheese - watch fat content).
- Fortified bread products.

You can also get your daily dose of vitamin D by spending 10-15 minutes a day in the sunshine with exposed face, arms & legs. Getting enough calcium and vitamin D is vital for bone health. Calcium can't absorb properly without sufficient vitamin D. Increasing your dairy intake to get more calcium is not the answer on its own as dairy is low in magnesium, and you need to balance both for strong bones. In fact, high calcium and low magnesium can lead to osteoporosis. Yes, I know, it's a bloody minefield!

You can still be sun-smart when you stroll out in the sunshine by wearing sunscreen. Studies have shown wearing sunscreen has little effect on your body's ability to absorb vitamin D. So slap it on, sit out in the sun, relax and let it do its goodness.

The other thing your bones love is exercise. I know you are going to say that they really don't, that everything hurts afterwards, your bones ache, you can actually hear your muscles screaming and you can barely sit down for a pee. I know it, been there, felt the burn! But that's just your bones and muscles telling you that you don't exercise enough, because if you did, they wouldn't be rebelling so much.

Yep, no let out clause.

If you factor in weight-bearing exercises at least 3 times a week. using free weights and resistance bands, your bones will love you for it.

Weight bearing exercises that stress the bones will aid the regeneration process and increase bone density. Your skeleton will silently thank you. I mean literally, no creaking or cracking every time you stand up or sit down.

FLEXING MUSCLE

There is truth in the adage 'you are what you eat'. And if you want to be strong into your later years you need to feed your muscles. You can achieve this by ensuring you eat enough protein, the building block of muscle, which is essential for keeping muscles healthy.

Aim to eat high protein food at least three times a day, and include:

- Lean meat.
- Chicken breast.
- Oily fish such as salmon and mackerel.
- Eggs.
- Cottage cheese.
- Almonds.
- Quinoa.
- Beans, like kidney beans and black beans.

Just as with your bones, your muscles need a daily healthy dose of vitamin D. There you have it, follow the advice for healthy bones and you get a bonus benefit of healthy muscles too.

Alongside this is the need for a regular exercise routine. Resistance exercise is best using a resistance band or hand weights. This will increase your muscle mass, strength, flexibility and balance.

HYDRATION

Keeping hydrated is an absolute necessity. I know you've heard it before - drink 8 glasses of water a day - but there's a very good reason why all proponents of good health keep banging on about it - your body needs it to function.

I know it's annoying, when trying to keep up the recommended water intake the more you need to pee, but it is so worth it when you consider the benefits the water is having on your bodily functions.

- It helps prevent kidneys stones.
- Regulates body temperature.
- Carries oxygen and nutrients to cells.
- Flushes out toxins when we pee.
- Breaks down food and aids digestion.
- Keeps skin hydrated and can reduce the appearance of wrinkles.

And remember, it's not just water that can rehydrate you, some foods are especially good for rehydration too:

- Cucumbers.
- Zucchini (courgettes).
- Tomatoes.
- Pineapple.

- Watermelon.
- Strawberries.

And then of course there's the usual lifestyle activities that will help clear brain fog:

- Regular sleep pattern.
- Daily exercise.
- Stress reducing activities.
- Quiet, relaxing time.
- Quit smoking.

We all love food, right? We love the taste of it, we love the cake, and the fish and chips from the chippy and the pizza. I think it's probably rare that people who have a plate of their favourite food put in front of them ever think "Well then... I should probably consider the nutritional content and balance of this food before I eat it".

In moderation, that's okay, but changing your relationship with food starts with acknowledging the main purpose of it. I feel I just need to drop in a little reminder about the reason we need to eat - to give our body the nutrients it needs to enable us to stay alive and function optimally - that's it, that's the reason our body needs food. It's important to enjoy your food but keep the balance and remember that not everything you eat and drink is good for you, regardless of how good it tastes.

I've said previously, you can't eat the same way as you did in your younger years. It's just a fact, you can't. Some foods will no longer agree with you. You must eat less if you want to maintain your weight and even less again if you want to lose it. We can all say "but I don't feel any different than I did years ago" - I say it all the time. But the fact is your body IS different, your hormones ARE changing, your metabolism IS slowing down, your food intolerances ARE going up. This means you need to be more mindful of what you eat and drink and make better choices.

Plan your meals to include protein at every meal, a small amount of carbohydrates (wholemeal or wholegrain bread, potato, brown rice) and plenty of vegetables in a variety of colours. Not because it looks pretty, but because the colour of food is an indication of the nutrients it contains. Remember to include enough calcium and iron rich foods in your day such as almonds, seeds, yoghurt, cottage cheese, kidney beans, black beans, lentils, lean meat, poultry, fish and leafy greens such as spinach.

Get used to checking food labels. Make it a habit. Make the majority of your food intake whole-foods - that is, food that has had minimal interference of processing or additives - and cut out foods that are clearly processed foods. Crowd out the bad stuff by gradually replacing it with a healthier option. Eat a high protein breakfast, snack only on cut up vegetables or small quantities of nuts and seeds. Watch your drinks, some are sugar-loaded!

No two women are alike when it comes to nutritional needs. However, balancing your macronutrients - your carbs, protein and fats - in the ratio required by your body as you get older, is the key. Your body does not metabolise food in the same way as it did when you were younger.

As your hormones change, your nutritional needs increase in some areas to compensate and decrease in others. And yes, you may need to take nutritional supplements, but only after you have been diagnosed deficient and preferably recommended by a healthcare professional.

Where possible you should get your nutrients, vitamins and minerals from your food. However, it's unrealistic to think it is always possible and especially as you get older, because even though you may have a wide and varied healthy diet, your body cannot absorb and distribute the nutrients as efficiently as it did when you were younger.

Self-care is more important than ever as you tick off the years and it is important to gain knowledge to recognise the subtle and not so subtle signs of change. Gain the knowledge you need to manage the changes yourself, or to guide you to when you should seek advice from a certified practitioner.

Health care professionals across the board agree that the symptoms of menopause and life beyond into old age can be successfully managed with education, lifestyle changes, healthy eating and exercise activities.

Knowledge is Power. Live Long, Live Healthy.

AFTERWORD

"Whatever happens, stay alive. Don't die before you're dead. Don't lose yourself, don't lose hope, don't lose direction.

Stay alive, with yourself, with every cell of your body, with every fiber of your skin.

Stay alive, learn, study, think, read, build, invent, create, speak, write, dream, design.

Stay alive, stay alive inside you, stay alive also outside, fill yourself with colors of the world, fill yourself with peace, fill yourself with hope.

Stay alive with joy.

There is only one thing you should not waste in life, and that's life itself."

~Virginia Woolf

About the Author

In 1994, following a period of emotional upheaval and notions of unfulfilled ambition, Karen Spence made a conscious decision to re-evaluate and reconstruct her life.

Karen was 36 when she enrolled in a full-time university degree. This marked the beginning of five transformative years on a journey of personal growth and self-discovery. Whilst attending university she continued to support herself working 28-hour weeks. She navigated the breakdown of her marriage and subsequent divorce, bought her own home and found love again with her husband Ivan. She graduated from university with Honours in 1997.

Karen and Ivan married in 1998 and faced new challenges. Efforts to conceive had failed and they endured the emotional roller-coaster of assisted fertility treatment, which was ultimately successful. In 1999, Karen was 41 years old when she and Ivan welcomed their daughter Rebecca.

She found herself once again wading through uncharted waters. This time, as a middle-aged, first-time mum experiencing the physical, mental and emotional challenges of post-birth, combined with the equally challenging and conflicting symptoms of perimenopause.

Karen Spence's journey is a testament to resilience, reinvention, and the power of pursuing life on your own terms, at any age.

Born in Manchester, UK, Karen grew up in a bustling household as the middle child of seven children. In 1975 at just 17 years old, Karen defied expectations and left secretarial college to enlist in the British Army where she enjoyed a rewarding 15-year career.

During the 15 years that followed she worked in the public sector in UK prior to emigrating to New Zealand and later to Australia, where she worked in central government roles in the respective countries.

In her mid-50s Karen elected early retirement to resurrect an earlier passion. Already a Certified Health & Weight Loss Coach, Karen further qualified as a Group Fitness Trainer and Aqua-aerobics Instructor. She created her own business to encourage and empower other middle-aged women to prioritise themselves and engage in meaningful self-care.

Now, with her first book, Karen dives into the unique challenges of the daily struggles associated with the stages of menopause and life beyond. She challenges women to step fearlessly into middle age, shattering outdated notions and proving that this time of life is just the beginning of new possibilities.

Her aim is to debunk societal myths and extinguish stereotypical attitudes and opinions of middle-aged women. She offers insights for women to reignite their enthusiasm, purpose and standing in today's society.

Her message is clear; this stage of your life can be your best yet, full of potential and opportunity - don't waste it.

Karen's passion is to encourage women to look to their future with confidence and purpose, keeping health and fitness, self-care and psychological self-preservation, at the heart of their journey.

REFERENCES

Alzheimer's Society. (2025). *Is dementia hereditary?* Retrieved from https://www.alzheimers.org.uk/about-dementia/is-dementia-hereditary

Australian Government Department of Health, Disability and Ageing. (2024, December 18). *Toxic chemicals in tobacco smoke.* Retrieved from https://www.health.gov.au/our-work/tobaccofacts/toxic-chemicals-in-tobacco-smoke

Bernhard, B., & Correa, R. (2024, September 6). *You're Not Overweight. Could You Still Develop Type 2 Diabetes?* Retrieved from HealthCentral: https://www.healthcentral.com/condition/type-2-diabetes/you-could-have-diabetes-while-healthy-weight-heres-how

Cancer Research UK. (n.d.). *Smoking, tobacco and cancer.* Retrieved from https://www.cancerresearchuk.org/about-cancer/causes-of-cancer/smoking-and-cancer

Key, K. (2022, May 18). *Midlife Depression in Women.* Retrieved from Psychology Today: https://www. psychologytoday.com/au/blog/counseling-keys/202205/ midlife-depression-in-women

Mayo Clinic. (2024, November 19). *Botox injections.* Retrieved from https://www.mayoclinic.org/tests-procedures/ botox/about/pac-20384658

Mishra, G., Barnes, I., Byrnes, E., Cavenagh, D., Dobson, A., Forder, P., . . . Byles, J. (2022). *Health and wellbeing for women in midlife: Findings from the Australian Longitudinal Study on Women's Health.* Report prepared for the Australian Government Department of Health.

Join the Community on Facebook

Midlife Mirth & Mayhem | Facebook
https://www.facebook.com/groups/3918878685108524/

ACKNOWLEDGEMENTS

To Rebecca and Veronique - thank you so much for your insight, feedback and suggestions in the early chapters of the book. It was very much appreciated.

NOTES

NOTES

NOTES

NOTES

Notes

NOTES

NOTES